THE
MEDICINE
OF THE
ANCIENT
EGYPTIANS

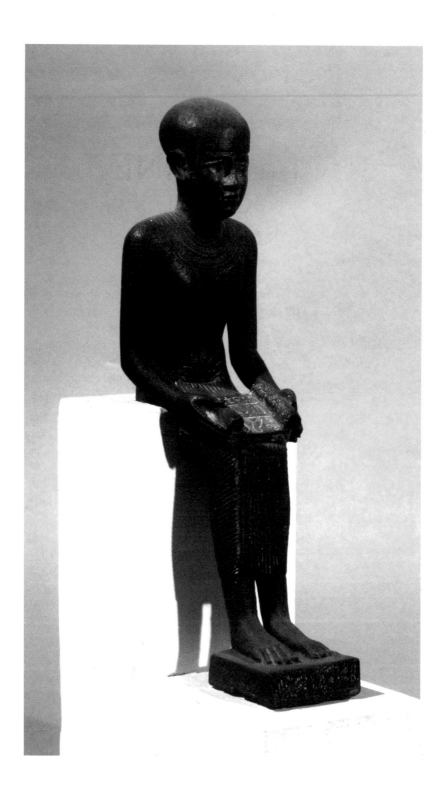

THE
MEDICINE
OF THE
ANCIENT
EGYPTIANS

1: SURGERY, GYNECOLOGY, OBSTETRICS, AND PEDIATRICS

Eugen Strouhal
Břetislav Vachala
Hana Vymazalová

The American University in Cairo Press
Cairo New York

Page ii: A bronze statue of Imhotep, a famous Egyptian sage and legendary physician. Imhotep was the architect of the earliest stone (step) pyramid of King Netjerikhet Djoser in Saqqara from the Third Dynasty. In later times, he was deified and venerated as the patron of medicine. (Ptolemaic to Roman Period, Egyptian Museum, Cairo [JE 38048], photo: M. Zemina)

The publisher wishes to thank Lisa Sabbahy for her kind help with the preparation of this book.

First published in English in 2014 by
The American University in Cairo Press
113 Sharia Kasr el Aini, Cairo, Egypt
420 Fifth Avenue, New York, NY 10018
www.aucpress.com

Copyright © 2010, 2014 by Charles University in Prague, Faculty of Arts

Originally published as *Lékařství starých Egypťanů I* in 2010 by Academia, Prague

Translated by Sean Mark Miller and Kateřina Millerová

Funding for this English edition was provided by the Program for the Development of Fields of Study at Charles University, No. 14: Archaeology of Non-European Areas, sub-program Research of Ancient Egyptian Civilization: Cultural and Political Adaptation of the North African Civilizations in Ancient History (5000 BC–AD 1000).

Illustrations © Hana Vymazalová, Jolana Malátková, 2010, 2014
Photography © Archive of the Czech Institute of Egyptology, Faculty of Arts, Charles University in Prague (Milan Zemina, Jan Brodský, Kamil Voděra); Manfred Bietak; Ladislava Horáčková; Mohamed Megahed; Andreas G. Nerlich; Eugen Strouhal; W. Michael Pahl; Sandro Vannini; Albert Zink; bpk/Ägyptisches Museum und Papyrussammlung, SMB/Margarete Büsing; Petrie Museum of Egyptian Archaeology, University College London; New York Academy of Medicine, 2010, 2014

Exclusive distribution outside Egypt and North America by I.B.Tauris & Co Ltd., 6 Salem Road, London, W2 4BU

Dar el Kutub No. 14522/13
ISBN 978 977 416 640 2

Dar el Kutub Cataloging-in-Publication Data

Strouhal, Eugen
    The Medicine of the Ancient Egyptians 1: Surgery, Gynecology, Obstetrics, and
    Pediatrics / Eugen Strouhal, Břetislav Vachala, and Hana Vymazalová.—Cairo: The American
University in Cairo Press, 2014
        p.   cm.
        ISBN: 978 977 416 640 2
        Medicine—Egypt— Antiquities
        610.932

1 2 3 4 5   18 17 16 15 14

Designed by Sally Boylan
Printed in Egypt

Contents

Preface

As a physician, archaeologist, anthropologist, and paleopathologist, I have been fascinated by ancient Egyptian medicine for almost half a century. My interest in it goes back to the time of my eight years of work in the Czechoslovak Institute of Egyptology of Charles University in Prague in the 1960s. After 1968, it further developed during my activities in the Náprstek Museum, a part of the National Museum in Prague. In 1986 and again in 1988, I gradually contacted two leading Czech publishing houses in Prague with the proposal of a monograph on ancient Egyptian medicine, which was then lacking in Czech or Slovak literature. The first proposal was rejected. The second attempt was made along with the Egyptologist Břetislav Vachala, who had offered for this purpose his translation of some medical papyri directly from the original ancient Egyptian texts into Czech. This enriched scientific project was not accepted either.

When I subsequently returned to Charles University in Prague (this time to its First Faculty of Medicine), my lectures on ancient Egyptian medicine became a regular part of the instruction of the history of medicine, and I have lectured on this topic there to this day. Not even then did my close cooperation with the Czech Institute of Egyptology end, as in the meantime the Institute had gained an excellent expert on ancient Egyptian science (in particular mathematics) in Hana Vymazalová, so that my colleague Dr. Vachala and I could successfully offer her participation in the research plan whose aim was to be a three-volume compendium, *The Medicine of the Ancient Egyptians*. We are presenting the first volume, dealing with ancient Egyptian surgery, gynecology, obstetrics, and pediatrics, with the wish that it address not only physicians but also all those interested in the history of ancient Egypt.

N.B.: The method of dating in this publication is based on *Ilustrovaná ency-klopedie starého Egypta* [An Illustrated Encyclopaedia of Ancient Egypt] (Verner, Bareš, and Vachala 1998).

Eugen Strouhal

Acknowledgments

The authors express their thanks to the New York Academy of Medicine; the Metropolitan Museum of Art in New York; the Petrie Museum of Egyptian Archaeology, University College London; and the Berlin State Museums, especially the Egyptian Museum and Papyrus Collection, for granting their rights for printing the papyri and objects from their collections.

Thanks are also owed to Dr. Filip Coppens for invaluable consultations in the translation of difficult passages from medicine and magic texts for chapter 4. We are grateful to Mohamed Megahed, Sandro Vannini, Dr. Michael Pahl, and Dr. Albert Zink for providing photographs at no charge and for their priceless assistance in the selection of the illustrations. We thank Jolana Malátková for providing several drawings. Our great thanks are owed to Fatma Abdel Moneim Megahed for inspiring consultations concerning the customs and superstitions in connection with pregnancy and childbirth in today's Upper Egypt.

This book has been created thanks to the support of the Czech Institute of Egyptology of Charles University in Prague and the Ministry of Education, Youth, and Sports of the Czech Republic. We are grateful for stimulating comments on the manuscript to our respected reviewers, Drs. Miloš Hájek and Jiří Janák.

We would also like to express our gratitude to Sean Mark Miller and Kateřina Millerová, who acquitted themselves in the challenging task of translating this book into English.

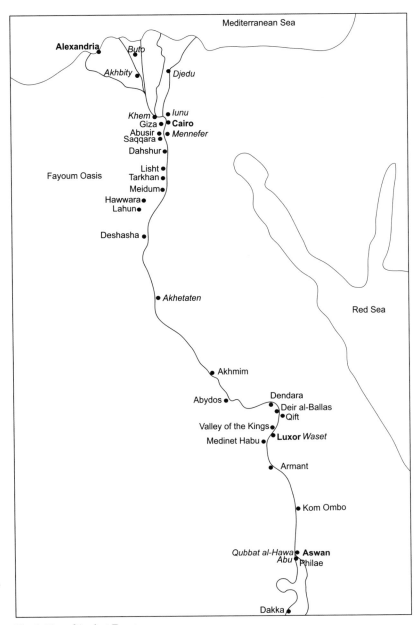

Fig. 1. Map of Ancient Egypt.

1

THE WISDOM OF THE AGES

Enchanted by the beauty of the monumental architecture and sculpture, the vividness and harmony of the colors of the mural reliefs, and the perfectly fashioned tiniest objects, we admire today the technical craft, patience, and taste of ancient Egyptians at a time when, with the exception of Mesopotamia, the rest of humanity lived in the Neolithic Age. Nevertheless, most of us do not realize that the Egyptians also excelled in other areas of human invention, especially in science. Egyptian medicine experienced a surprisingly rapid development as early as the Old Kingdom and preserved its good reputation both at home and abroad even in the following centuries. It is proved, for example, by a relief from the tomb of Nebamun, a personal physician of King Amenhotep II, depicting a medical consultation with foreigners. Nebamun here is providing a curative drink to a Syrian nobleman, who had had to undergo a long journey in order to acquire relief from his illness (fig. 2). We are also informed of the high level of knowledge and the great number of Egyptian physicians by the famous authors of pre-Classical and Classical Greece.

Homer mentions Egypt in *The Odyssey* as a land "where fertile soil produces the greatest share of medicines, many good in mixtures, [but also] many harmful . . . every man there is a physician and understands [knows] more than men elsewhere" (Homer, *Odyssey* IV, §229–32). The father of ancient historiography Herodotus, on the other hand, was fascinated by the

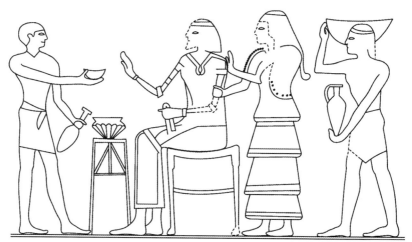

Fig. 2. A relief from the tomb of Nebamun, a court physician of King Amenhotep II, shows Nebamun giving a curative drink to a Syrian nobleman. This scene suggests that the fame of Egyptian medicine attracted the sick from surrounding lands. (Eighteenth Dynasty, tomb of Nebamun [TT 17] at Dra Abu al-Naga, drawing: H. Vymazalová after Wreszinski 1923, Pl. 115)

high level of specialization of the Egyptian physicians: "Medicine with them is divided so that everyone is a physician for one disease and not for more diseases. Physicians are everywhere there. Some are eye doctors, others heal the head, others teeth, and still others the stomach and others invisible diseases" (Herodotus, *History* II, §84–85).

A number of ancient philosophers, scholars, and physicians expressed thanks in their autobiographies for knowledge acquired in practice in Egypt. The study of medicine in the land on the banks of the Nile meant for them the highest qualification and recommendation. Egyptian medicine is mentioned with great respect by ancient authors in their works (for example, Diodorus of Sicily, *Bibliotheca Historica* I: 82; Pliny the Elder, *Natural History* XXIX: 1). It is indisputable that ancient Egyptian medicine influenced the advancement of medicine in cultures around the Aegean Sea, but primarily in Greece, where its uninterrupted continuation through the medicine of the Roman Empire eventually became European medicine. That could be a reason for the interest in the scientific beginnings of medical knowledge, so important for life, for which we are indebted to the ancient Egyptians.

Modern authors of books and specialized articles on Egyptian medicine admire its breadth and depth and appreciate that, while preserving magical healing methods of the previous prehistoric period, it matured with the accumulation of rational knowledge acquired in everyday experience (von Deines, Grapow, and Westendorf 1958; Ghalioungui and el-Dawakhly 1965; Kamal 1967; Leca 1971; Ghalioungui 1973, 1983; Estes 1989; Bardinet 1995; Nunn 1996; Westendorf 1992, 1999; Stephan 2001; Allen 2005). As the first in the ancient world, medicine in ancient Egypt formed a comprehensive system that can be deciphered thanks to the collection of thirteen medical texts found so far.

The Texts—Key to Ancient Egyptian Medicine

Egyptian medical papyri are unparalleled in other cultures. They would not have emerged without the early creation of a writing system in the Predynastic and Archaic periods on the one hand, and the invention of a suitable writing medium—papyrus—on the other. The strips of the inner pith of the stem of the aquatic plant papyrus sedge *(Cyperus papyrus)*, growing in the swamps on the banks of the Nile and in the network of its branching canals, cut lengthwise, were placed both side by side and across at right angles on a hard surface and briskly beaten by the stone or wooden mallets used at the time. Having released the juices, the strips bonded together and created white sheets, similar in size to our paper, on which the scribes wrote with a reed brush dipped in black or red ink. Along with the system of writing, this created a means for the long-term recording not only of the administrative issues of everyday life or literary compositions, but also of scientific knowledge, whose preservation no longer depended solely on oral transmission.

The papyrus stalks were, however, not used to make books like those we know today. Sheets of a height of approximately 40 cm (or 20 cm) were glued together to form a roll of the necessary length (Parkinson and Quirke 1995, 16), which was fixed at each end onto a wooden rod, so that when it was being read it could be unrolled and simultaneously rolled onto the other rod. The scribes wrote their documents in the hieratic script, the cursive version of the hieroglyphic script reserved only for monumental inscriptions (fig. 3), usually right to left, in columns of text of various widths from top to bottom. The papyrus scrolls, which the Egyptians kept in wooden containers or stowed in pigeonholes in the walls of the libraries of the time, could be preserved for numerous centuries thanks to favorable climatic conditions, with predominantly dry and hot weather. The finds of medical papyri are a unique, and truly the most important, source of our knowledge on ancient Egyptian medicine. Such sources are lacking in other cultures.

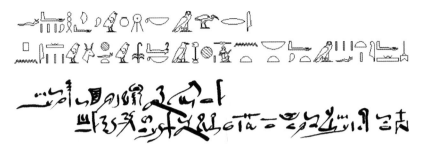

Fig. 3. The hieratic text of a part of the Edwin Smith Papyrus and its hieroglyphic transcription: "When you discover a wound whose flesh is missing and the edges are separated from any human limb, you must follow these instructions." (Smith 47)

Both makers and readers of papyri were physicians, who, thanks to their ability to read and write, ranked among the educated (literate) class of Egyptian society—the scribes, the intelligentsia of the time. Some specialists have considered a possible relationship or link between the physicians and embalmers, from whom the physicians allegedly learned the anatomy of the human body and of diseased organs. This hypothesis was evoked by ignorance, by a confusion of modern medical autopsy and ancient Egyptian mummification, which had hardly anything in common (Strouhal 1994). The embalmers' task was to remove the internal organs from the dead body, and sometimes also the brain from the cranium. They performed this unappealing work roughly, sometimes even loutishly. Having sliced the left hypochondrium open, they cut or tore the organs from the abdominal cavity almost blindly, only by touch, and after they tore the diaphragm, they cut the organs from the thoracic cavity as well. In accordance with the ideas of that time concerning the composition and functioning of the human organism, the only organ they had to leave in the cavity was the heart, which contained in itself the identity of the person. Both professions were under the patronage of various gods—medicine under the protection of the goddess Sekhmet or Serket (Selket) (figs. 4, 5), mummification under the protection of the god Anubis (fig. 6). Members of the first comprised the peak within the intelligentsia, enjoying the respect and admiration of the society. The others were craftsmen, and for their dirty and horrifying work the rest rather abhorred them and sometimes even stoned them, although more figuratively than in reality.

Medical papyri can be considered as everyday manuals for the rational decision-making and practical action of physicians, whatever their special

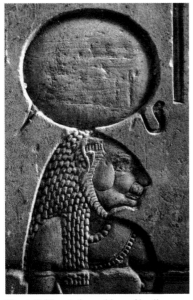

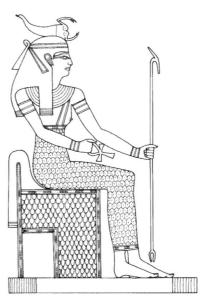

Fig. 4. Sekhmet, the goddess of healing, depicted as a woman with the head of a lioness and a solar disc on top of her head. Her name means 'the Mighty One.' (Ptolemaic to Roman Period, Dakka, photo: M. Megahed)

Fig. 5. Serqet, in the form of a woman with a scorpion on her head, was associated with motherhood and child care, but she also protected people from dangerous animals, scorpions, and snakes. (Nineteenth Dynasty, tomb of Queen Nefertari [QV 66] in the Valley of the Queens, drawing: J. Malátková)

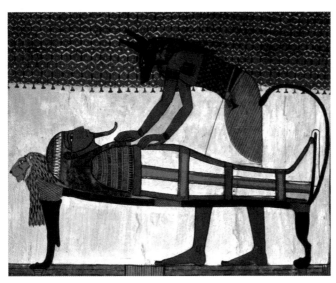

Fig. 6. Isis's guardian, the jackal-headed Anubis, was the god of mummification, death, and resurrection. (Nineteenth Dynasty, tomb of Sennedjem [TT 1] at Deir al-Medina, photo: M. Zemina)

activity's focus was. They were a guideline for them according to which they healed their patients. We therefore think that the papyri were copied abundantly, although no exact duplicates of any of the individual medical papyri have been found as of yet. Their content gradually became set and was considered holy.

Their supernatural origin or divine inspiration was even believed in. Hence the text on the Papyrus Berlin 3038 (163a) states that its scroll "was found in a library with old treatises and documents at the feet of Anubis in Khem (Letopolis in Greek) at the time of His Majesty King of Upper and Lower Egypt Den . . . ," hence in the First Dynasty. We can find a very similar claim also in the Ebers Medical Papyrus (856a).

The existence of medical papyri seems to have been proved already during the Old Kingdom by an inscription in the tomb of the chief architect Washptah from the time of King Neferirkare (Fifth Dynasty). When during the king's inspection this dignitary suffered a stroke or an injury (Picardo 2010), the king had a library with papyri brought so that the physician could attempt to revive the stricken man (Strudwick 2005, 318–19). In the papyrus from the British Museum in London (BM 10059, 25), it is written that this "book was found at night when it fell to the court of the temple in Qift [Coptos in Greek], as the secret knowledge of this goddess [= Isis], (written) by the hand of a lector of this temple . . ." As a miraculous find, it was taken to King Khufu (Fourth Dynasty), more famous under the Greek name of Cheops, who was the builder of the largest pyramid in Giza. This indirectly proves the early existence of at least some medical texts.

The papyri represented not only authority, but at the same time the shield of the physicians in case of an unsuccessful treatment. Diodorus put it well: "If they [the physicians] follow the instructions of the holy book and still cannot save the ill, they are released of any prosecution. If they do something against the prescriptions, they will be sentenced to death" (*Bibliotheca Historica* I, 82: 3, 281). As practical handbooks, medical papyri were not intended for the systematic enumeration and categorization of the medical knowledge of the time. Through a careful study of them, we can find, assemble, and reconstruct various aspects and conceptions that prove the existence of the earliest medical system of the ancient world (Stephan 2001, 259–62).

The second function of the medical scrolls was their use in teaching the young pupils medicine. They studied, like the students of other fields, in the 'houses of life,' which were not laboratories or hospitals but more like libraries and scriptoria. In their walls, rolled papyrus scrolls were available to the students. They read them repeatedly; they might have learned to recite them by heart, just as to this day pupils of Qur'anic schools learn the *suras* (chapters) of the Qur'an.

Individual medical papyri have diverse contents. Didactic texts, collections of instructions, directions for practice, and similar things alternate with specialized essays, sometimes taken from other cited treatises, which have not been preserved.

It cannot be expected that we will find in the papyri the names and descriptions of diseases (nosological units), which modern medicine has elucidated only since the nineteenth century. The titles or the descriptions of the examinations mention only the symptoms that are to be treated.

Whereas the cause of the appearance of wounds and injuries was usually clear, the Egyptians generally sought the origin of internal illnesses with the pantheon of their gods, whose favor needed to be won by magical–ritual means, especially sacrifices. Nevertheless, health problems could also be caused by various demons, which had to be expelled from the sick. It is for this reason that magical enchantments and practices with a magical effect are mixed in the papyri with rational methods and empirically proven medicines.

A Selection of Monographs on Ancient Egyptian Medicine

The first Czech translation of the Smith Papyrus was made by the founder of Czech Egyptology, František Lexa, in collaboration with the surgeon Arnold Jirásek (Lexa and Jirásek 1941).

In world literature, ancient Egyptian medicine has received attention at least since the publication of the Ebers Papyrus (Ebers 1875). In the past twenty-five years, several professional and popular science monographs have been published, of which we can mention a few examples, starting with a book by an American pharmacologist dealing with Egyptian healers, patients, surgery, internal medicine, and medications (Estes 1989). Diseases of various body parts and their treatment were analyzed mainly in the works written by a great German Egyptologist (Westendorf 1992, 1999). A new French translation of the Ebers, Hearst, and Berlin 3038 papyri, the Kahun and other gynecological papyri, as well as the London and Brooklyn papyri, was published with a commentary and analysis of medical theories (Bardinet 1995). An English medical scientist who had studied the basics of the ancient Egyptian language for a quarter of a century wrote a well-designed and richly illustrated book, using a style comprehensible to the general public (Nunn 1996). An Egyptian specialist in industrial medicine and a major-general in the Egyptian army gathered pieces of knowledge from different branches of medicine, especially occupational (Ebeid 1999). The relation between magic and rationality in ancient Egyptian disease conception and therapeutic practice, discussed by Egyptian and German authors (Kolta and Schwarzmann-Schafhauser 2000), was strongly criticized (Quack 2003). Another German physician and Egyptologist recognized systems in the order of the cases in the Ebers Papyrus and studied the cases in the Edwin Smith Papyrus in terms of pathology, pathophysiology, and medical history and translated them anew into German (Stephan 2001).

The catalogue of an exhibition on the art of Egyptian medicine contains the latest English translation of the Smith Papyrus (Allen 2005). Ancient Egyptian medicine from the perspective of an Egyptian author was based mainly on domestic sources (Faied 2006). Eighteen magical and medical papyri, the word for magic *(heka)*, and the main types of pathological changes were described by a Portuguese author (Veiga 2009).

The *Medicine of the Ancient Egyptians* Program

The first volume of the commented translations of the medical texts, *The Medicine of the Ancient Egyptians: Surgery, Gynecology, Obstetrics, and Pediatrics*, contains a translation of the Edwin Smith Papyrus, which stands out for its almost exclusively empirical and rational knowledge. It is complemented by surgical passages in the conclusion of the Ebers Papyrus. Women's illnesses and obstetrics are included in the Kahun Papyrus and Papyrus Carlsberg VIII; the care of women and children can also be found in selected passages from the Ebers Papyrus, from the papyri from the Ramesseum, and from the museums in London and Berlin. We have also considered the so-called *Book for Mother and Child*, which constitutes an excellent example of the magic used for the treatment and protection of women and their babies.

The second volume, *Internal Medicine*, will cover a translation of the main part of the Ebers Papyrus, the Hearst Papyrus, and excerpts from other texts. Physicians in ancient Egypt, not knowing the functions of the internal organs, treated the evident symptoms of their diseases by empirically tested means, which were mingled with magical–ritual methods.

The third volume, *Physicians, Diseases, and Treatment*, will closely build on both of the previous volumes. Besides the knowledge from the papyri, it will also utilize other literary and archaeological sources. It will discuss the physicians and their assistants, medical hierarchy (titles), specializations, remedies and their application, and so on. It will summarize the anatomical knowledge from which the physiological and pathophysiological conception of health and disease then grew. Attention will also be paid to the diseases existing then, namely congenital, degenerative, infectious, parasitic, neo-plastic, and others. It will also deal with smaller fields such as eye, ear, nose, throat, skin, and dental medicine and prosthetics. It will cover ancient Egypt-ian pharmacopeia—medicines from the plant, animal, and mineral king-doms—and discuss the efficacy of these medicines. Insufficient hygiene and its consequences, culminating in the appearance of the first epidemics, will be included as well. In the conclusion, the evidence of the transfer of knowl-edge from Egyptian medicine to Greek and hence also to European medicine will be considered.

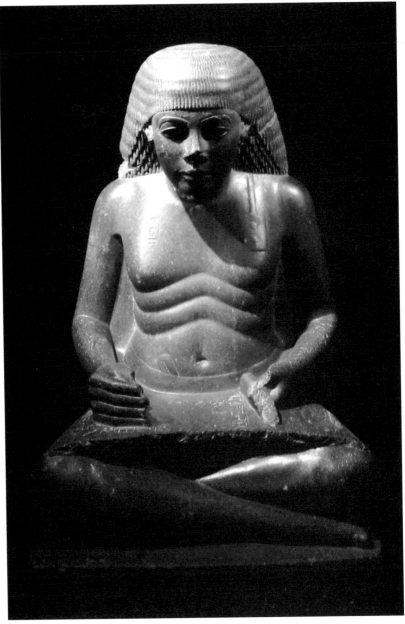

Fig. 7. This statue of Amenhotep, son of Hapu, is the prototype of an Egyptian scribe, a representative of the educated elite, in a typical seated position with a scroll unrolled on his lap. Every physician had to become a scribe first. (Eighteenth Dynasty, Luxor Museum [J 4], Egyptian Museum, Cairo [JE 44862], photo: M. Megahed)

2

PAPYRUS SCROLLS OF THE
EGYPTIAN PHYSICIANS

The texts that have been preserved from ancient Egypt represent only an infinitesimal fragment of all the scientific scrolls written back then, stored and studied in the libraries of ancient Egyptian temples. The larger or smaller fragments of papyri that have escaped the ravages of time and survived to this day are carefully stored in the collections of the world's museums. They capture sundry medical cases and reflect the real and oftentimes painful hardships of the population of the famous land on the banks of the Nile, in strong contrast with the sublime and lofty feeling left on visitors by the majestic stone temples and monumental tombs built by those people.

The following synopsis captures the essential information on the individual papyri. The texts are organized roughly by age from the earliest to the latest, although it is naturally impossible to determine their date with absolute certainty. The only exception in the chronological order is the *Book for Mother and Child* (Papyrus Berlin 3027), which we have attached at the very end, since it is not a classic medical text. In many cases, the precise provenance of the texts is not known, because some papyri were purchased by experts on the antiquities market and the records of their origin are missing. Besides a brief overview of the contents of the texts, the basic publications and translations are listed here.

All of the texts we will deal with are written in hieratic script and come from the time of the Middle and New Kingdoms. We also know later medical papyri written in demotic, some of which contain cases related to our topic (demotic papyri from London, Leiden, the Brooklyn Museum, and the Crocodilopolis Papyrus), but in this publication we have limited ourselves to the earlier texts, reflecting the knowledge and practice of the ancient Egyptian physicians without influences from abroad, which are often evident in the later texts from all of the scientific branches.

Kahun Papyrus
Origin of the text
The gynecological papyrus was one of the many papyrus fragments that were found in April and November 1889 during the excavations of the British archaeologist Flinders Petrie in Lahun, in the pyramid town mistakenly called Kahun. The text was written at the end of the Middle Kingdom, perhaps during the reign of Amenemhat III (Twelfth Dynasty), whose twenty-ninth year of reign was recorded on the reverse of the papyrus. Since its discovery, the papyrus has formed part of the collections of the Petrie Museum of Egyptian Archaeology at University College London.

Contents
The text covers three sheets and is written in the hieratic script. As the papyrus has been significantly damaged, some cases are difficult to understand, because they have been preserved only in part. The text includes thirty-four cases, dealing with various topics related to women.

Publication
Griffith 1898, 5–11, Pl. 5–6: a facsimile of hieratic texts, hieroglyphic transcription, translation into English, commentary.
von Deines, Grapow, and Westendorf 1958: translation into German.
Stevens 1975: translation into English.
Bardinet 1995, 221–29, 437–43: translation into French, commentary.
Collier and Quirke 2004, 58–64: translation into English.

Ramesseum Papyri
Origin of the text
These papyri were found in 1896 by the British archaeologist James Edward Quibell in the district of the monumental mortuary temple of the famous pharaoh Ramesses II, which is called the Ramesseum today. In one of the storage areas beyond the temple, a shaft tomb was discovered and in it a wooden box with seventeen papyrus scrolls. According to Alan Gardiner, the shaft

most likely served as a burial place of a magician or healer, which was implied also by other finds from his funerary equipment. The mention of Amenemhat III (Twelfth Dynasty) in one of the papyri makes it possible to date the texts approximately to the period of the Thirteenth Dynasty. The papyri are currently deposited in the Ashmolean Museum of Art and Archaeology, University of Oxford.

Contents

Three of the papyri have medical content. Papyrus III includes sixty-five cases in two sections (A, B), which deal with various illnesses of, for example, eyes, women, and children. Papyrus IV contains a total of forty-five cases in five sections (A–E) with various topics, including women's and children's medicine. In most of these cases, however, the treatment is magical. Papyrus V is less magical and more practical; it deals with various general illnesses and blood-vessel and muscle ailments.

Publication

Gardiner 1955: hieratic text.
Barns 1956: hieroglyphic transcription, commentary.
von Deines, Grapow, and Westendorf 1958: translation into German.
Bardinet 1995, 446, 451, 454, 466–75: translation into French.

Edwin Smith Papyrus
Origin of the text

Nothing is known of the origin of the text or its discovery. It is supposed that it comes from the tomb of a physician in the Theban necropolis, and it is possible that it was uncovered along with the Ebers Papyrus, which is very similar in script and language, and perhaps also with the mathematical Rhind Papyrus. The Edwin Smith Papyrus was purchased in Luxor by the American Edwin Smith from an Egyptian trader and consular agent, Mustafa Agha, in 1862. After Smith's death in 1906, his daughter offered the papyrus to the New-York Historical Society; today it is deposited in the New York Academy of Medicine. It is 4.7 m long and 32 cm wide.

Contents

The text covers seventeen sheets on the recto and five sheets on the verso; the majority is written in hieratic script, which can be dated approximately to the Sixteenth–Seventeenth Dynasties. On the basis of certain linguistic curiosities, some experts believe that the original text came from the Old Kingdom.

The majority of the text is nevertheless written in Classical Egyptian, and it is possible that the text at the time of its writing merely bore quite normal signs of archaizing. The dominant part of the text describes surgical cases related to the upper part of the body; on the verso, we find one case dealing with menstruation.

Publication
Breasted 1930: facsimile, translation into English, commentary.
Ebbell 1939: medical commentary.
Lexa and Jirásek 1941: translation into Czech.
von Deines, Grapow, and Westendorf 1958: translation into German.
Westendorf 1966: translation into German.
Žába 1968, 157–58: translation of Case 4 into Czech.
Bardinet 1995, 493–522, 453: translation into French.
Allen 2005: color photography, translation into English.

Ebers Papyrus
Origin of the text
The papyrus was purchased by Edwin Smith in Luxor in 1862. We do not have precise information on its discovery, but it was supposedly found with a mummy in a tomb at the cemetery in Asasif on the west bank of the Nile in Luxor. In 1872, the papyrus was purchased by the professor of Egyptology George Ebers and today can be found in the University Library in Leipzig (Voß 2009). The papyrus comprises 110 sheets and is the longest preserved medical papyrus (with a length of 20.23 m). It is dated to the ninth year of the reign of Amenhotep I (Eighteenth Dynasty).

Contents
The papyrus records an extensive collection of 877 medical cases with diverse foci. There are internal, skin, urinary, surgical, and other cases here; it describes the ways to heal headaches, burns, and bites from poisonous animals as well. It also contains women's problems and cases of childhood illnesses.

Publication
Ebers 1875: facsimile, Egyptian–Latin dictionary.
Joachim 1890: translation into German.
Wreszinski 1913: hieroglyphic transcription.
Bryan 1930: translation into English.

Ebbell 1937: translation into English.
von Deines, Grapow, and Westendorf 1958: translation into German.
Ghalioungui 1987: translation into English.
Bardinet 1995, 251–373, 443–51: translation into French.

Hearst Papyrus
Origin of the text
This papyrus was brought by one of the villagers from Deir al-Ballas in Upper Egypt to an expedition from the University of California led by George Reisner in 1901. The text was named after the American patron Phoebe Hearst, who financed Reisner's research. The papyrus may have been written during the reign of Thutmose III (Eighteenth Dynasty). Today, it is the property of the University of California, Berkeley.

Contents
The papyrus is made up of eighteen pages divided into 260 paragraphs. The cases deal with various problems, including digestive and urinary; they further concern blood, blood vessels, hair, bones, and bites. They also include a number of incantations. Roughly one hundred of the total number of 260 cases have parallels in the Ebers Papyrus.

Publication
Reisner 1905: hieratic text and a brief description of the contents.
von Deines, Grapow, and Westendorf 1958: translation into German.
Bardinet 1995, 375–408: translation into French.

London Papyrus BM 10059
Origin of the text
Nothing is known of the origin of the papyrus. Until 1860, it belonged to the Royal Institute in London; later it became the property of the British Museum in London. It is a palimpsest, a scroll whose original text was scraped off to make room for another text. In the original text on the papyrus, it is possible to recognize a date near the reign of Tutankhamun (Eighteenth Dynasty), which dates the text roughly to the middle of the New Kingdom.

Contents
The text covers nineteen sheets with twenty-five medical cases and thirty-six magical incantations. Several cases are related to women's problems; seventeen cases have parallels in the Ebers Papyrus.

Publication

Wreszinski 1912: translation into German.
von Deines, Grapow, and Westendorf 1958: translation into German.
Bardinet 1995, 483–92: translation into French.

Papyrus Carlsberg VIII

Origin of the text

Nothing is known of the origin of the text; it most likely comes from the Nineteenth or Twentieth Dynasty but was probably copied from an earlier model with a date closer to the Kahun Papyrus. It is the property of the Carlsberg Foundation and is housed at the Egyptological Institute of the University of Copenhagen.

Contents

The manuscript differs on the verso and recto. The recto is significantly damaged. The verso contains seven cases written on two sheets. The preserved cases are related to the determination of pregnancy, the sex of an unborn child, and a woman's fertility. Parallels are known from the Papyrus Berlin 3038 and the Kahun Papyrus.

Publication

Iversen 1939: translation into English.
von Deines, Grapow, and Westendorf 1958: translation into German.
Bardinet 1995, 442, 451, 452, 453, 465: translation into French.

Papyrus Berlin 3038

Origin of the text

Nothing is known of the origin of the text, but both the textual style and the script correspond to the period of the Nineteenth Dynasty. The papyrus was acquired by Giuseppe Passalacqua in Saqqara and in 1827 became part of the collection of antiquities of King Frederick William IV of Prussia, intended for the museum in Berlin.

Contents

In three places, the text mentions the author whose name (or function) was Netjerhetepu ('who soothes the god'). The text covers twenty-one sheets on the recto and three sheets on the verso. Most cases are an analogy of the cases from the Ebers Papyrus. Cases 13–18 deal with breast diseases, Case 192 contains a contraceptive agent, and Cases 193–199 describe the methods of determining a pregnancy, parallels for which are known only from the Kahun Papyrus and the Papyrus Carlsberg.

Publication
Brugsch 1863, 101–20, pl. LXXXV–CVII: facsimile of the hieratic text, commentary.
Wreszinski 1909: translation into German.
von Deines, Grapow, and Westendorf 1958: translation into German.
Bardinet 1995, 409–37, 451–53: translation into French.

Chester Beatty Papyri
Origin of the text
These papyri belonged to the family archive of the scribe Kenherkhepeshef from the Nineteenth Dynasty and remained in the holdings of his offspring for more than one hundred years. In 1928, they were found in the tomb chapel No. 1165 at Deir al-Medina on the west bank of the Nile in Luxor (Parkinson and Quirke 1995, 62–64). They afterward came into the holdings of Alfred Chester Beatty, a wealthy British industrialist, collector, and philanthropist, and later were deposited in the British Museum in London (BM 10685, 10686, 10687, 10688, 10695).

Contents
The five papyri known as Chester Beatty V–VIII and XV contain medical texts. On Papyrus V, we find an incantation against headache; Papyrus VI offers an overview of the healing of diseases of the rectum; the incantations on Papyrus VII were to aid against scorpion stings. Papyrus VIII contains many magical incantations and one prescription. The only preserved sheet of Papyrus XV includes two prescriptions against thirst.

Publication
Gardiner 1935: translation into English.
Jonckheere 1947: translation into French.
von Deines, Grapow, and Westendorf 1958: translation into German.
Bardinet 1995, 455–61, 478–79: translation into French.

Book for Mother and Child (Papyrus Berlin 3027)
Origin of the text
Nothing is known of the origin of the papyrus. In 1843, it was bought by Karl Richard Lepsius from the collection of Giovanni d'Athanasi; Sotheby's Auction

Catalogue (No. 961) at the same time said that they were papyrus scrolls found in Thebes and Memphis. The paleography indicates that the manuscript is contemporary with the Ebers Papyrus.

Contents
The scroll was composed of six sheets of high-quality papyrus, glued together. The text covered both sides of the papyrus and contained a total of twenty-one incantations and instructions for the protection of a woman and child. The text was evidently written down by two different scribes, each of whose handwriting is easily distinguished.

Publication
Erman 1901: translation into German.
Lexa 1923, II, 31–40: translation of twelve selected incantations into Czech.
Bardinet 1995, 477–78: translation into French.
Yamazaki 2003: translation into German.

3

ANCIENT EGYPTIAN SURGERY

W e have decided to begin the first volume of *The Medicine of the Ancient Egyptians* with a discussion of ancient Egyptian surgery. It represents the peak of the ancient physicians' attempts to investigate the complex mechanism of the human body with a rational, scientific approach to the diagnosis and prognosis of injuries and other pathological changes on the body surface. The Egyptians achieved this at the time when the world around them, with the exception of Mesopotamia, lived in the cultures of the Late Neolithic and Early Bronze Period.

The experience of ancient Egyptian surgeons and healers stemmed mainly from war wounds (fig. 9), but also, for example, from frequent injuries at construction sites as well as elsewhere at work. In contrast to internal illnesses, the cause of external illnesses was in most cases evident, so that treatment methods were usually rational and effective, and it was not necessary to strive to appease forces hostile to humanity by means of magic, as is often the case in other branches of ancient Egyptian medicine.

Medical Texts Dealing with Surgery
Surgical cases may be found in the two most famous medical papyri preserved from ancient Egypt, namely the Edwin Smith Papyrus and the Ebers Papyrus. The former is entirely devoted to surgery, specifically the treatment of injuries of the upper body, which is the reason that it is sometimes called the "Surgical

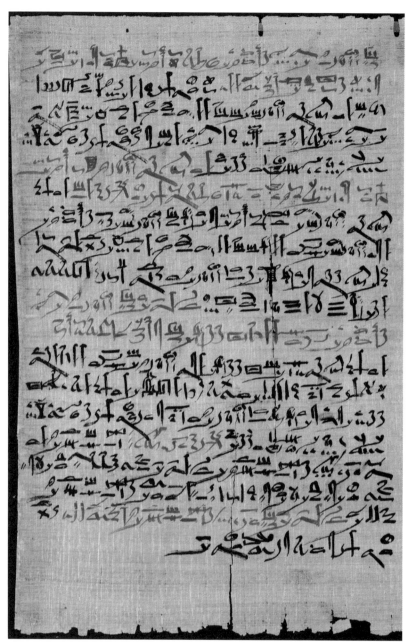

Fig. 8. The Edwin Smith Surgical Papyrus, also known as the Book of Wounds, has been preserved in good condition, and the hieratic script is still easily legible. (Fifteenth Dynasty, courtesy of the New York Academy of Medicine Library)

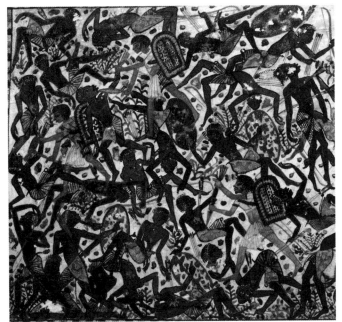

Fig. 9. From the earliest periods, Egyptian physicians and healers acquired extensive experience with wounds from military campaigns and battles. This box from Tutankhamun's treasure depicts a raging battle with many wounded fighters. (Eighteenth Dynasty, Egyptian Museum, Cairo [JE 61467], photo: S. Vannini)

Papyrus." It is one of the most valuable sources for the research into and understanding of ancient Egyptian medicine (Quack 2003). The Ebers Papyrus contains a wide range of cases of diverse medical topics, and its conclusion has a group of cases describing "knife treatment," surgical procedures for the treatment of ulcers and swellings.

An overview of the texts and respective cases dealing with surgery is given in table 1. The essential information on the particular medical texts, specifying their age, the circumstances and context of their discovery, their current location, and the list of earlier publications and translations, is given in chapter 2. More detailed information on the content of the texts appears below.

Table 1. Synopsis of surgical texts

Papyrus	Number of Cases	Topic
Edwin Smith	48	wounds and other illnesses
Ebers	16	tumors, cysts, infections, hernias, hematomas, ascites
Total number of cases	64	

The Edwin Smith Papyrus (fig. 8), the most famous ancient Egyptian medical papyrus, was named after its original owner, the American antique dealer Edwin Smith (1822–1906) (Dawson, Uphill, and Bierbrier 1995, 395). The Edwin Smith papyrus was first scientifically covered and issued in two exquisite volumes in 1930 by the American Egyptologist James H. Breasted, whose medical consultant was Dr. Arno Luckhardt (Breasted 1930). Since then it has been the object of interesting Egyptological as well as medical studies (recently: Brawarski 2001, 2004; Hofmann 2008) up to the most recent commented translation by James P. Allen (2005, 70–115). It is also worth mentioning the Czech translation of this papyrus by František Lexa, who cooperated in the publication with the renowned surgeon Arnold Jirásek (Lexa and Jirásek 1941).

The text was recorded on both sides of the papyrus by one scribe, with the exception of the last twenty-seven lines on the reverse. More authors are implied by the different lengths of the individual cases—with some, many details are presented, with others only the basic facts—or sporadic omission of some parts of the procedures—examination, prognosis, treatment, or explanatory notes. The text was written down somewhere in the area of Waset (Thebes in Greek, today's Luxor), and it was probably deposited in the temple library or in the tomb of its last owner. Nevertheless, the experienced scribe copying the original model, which was possibly as much as three hundred years old, made some mistakes. Judging by the results of a linguistic study of the text, it is unlikely that the model would have come from the Old Kingdom as some Egyptologists had believed, even directly from the quill of Imhotep, the venerated sage who lived during the reign of the sovereign Netjerikhet Djoser (Third Dynasty) and was later identified with the Greek god of medicine, Asclepius.

The text on the recto of the Edwin Smith Papyrus contains a specialized, methodical discussion on the treatment of wounds that were often incurred, especially on construction sites or in wars, and with which the physicians had extensive experience. The descriptions of the injuries and their treatment have been arranged systematically beginning from the head. In the copying, the scribe reached Case 48, the contusion of a thoracic vertebra, which he for some reason did not finish, abandoning the text in the middle of the case and in mid-sentence. The text is the preserved part—roughly the first quarter—of an extensive surgical treatise, the oldest of the medical papyri, containing rational, empirical knowledge of the ancient Egyptian physicians on the diagnosis and treatment of wounds. Some scholars call this text "Book of Wounds" ("Wundenbuch": Grapow 1958; Pahl 1985–86). Only in one case (No. 9) is the causal treatment complemented by a recitation of a traditional magical incantation. In this surprisingly modern character, the papyrus distinctly and uniquely differs from all the other medical treatises of ancient Egypt, as well as the Near East.

The preserved part of the papyrus orders the cases from the top of the head (the cranial vault, 1–8) through the forehead (9), eyebrows (10), nose (11–14), face (15–17), the temporal area (18–22), ear (23), lower jaw (24–25), lip (26), chin (27), throat (28), cervical vertebrae (29–33), clavicle (34–35), humerus (36–38), chest (39–41, 45–47), and ribs (42–44), all the way to a thoracic vertebra (48). It essentially corresponds to the order of contemporary anatomy. Within each division, the cases are sometimes listed according to their severity; at other times, the cases with good, uncertain, and bad prognoses alternate at random.

The titles of individual cases ("Instructions on . . .") are mostly written in red, just like some important sentences or even entire passages. The title of the case is followed by a description of the wound, determination of the diagnosis, the treatment method, and possible explanatory notes ("Concerning . . ."). A component of the diagnosis is the statement of the physician that it is "a disease that I will treat" (thirty prognoses), "a disease that I will contend with" (eight prognoses), or "a disease that nothing can be done about" (fourteen prognoses). Most cases have been described precisely and objectively, and the treatment is rational (with the exception of two mentions in the explanatory notes and in the incantations in Cases 8 and 9). The patient is always labeled by a word with the meaning of 'man, someone,' which in Egyptian is a general label for any person, including women and children. To a significant extent, men were exposed to wounds more often than women or children. Twice a reference is made to an unpreserved medical treatise, "Dealing with Wounds" (in Cases 5 and 41), and once to another unknown treatise, "The Skill of an Embalmer" (Case 19).

The presentation of the treatment method with a list of the possible treatment procedures or medicines is followed by the author's or copier's commentary ("explanations," after Allen 2005), whose aim is to clarify for the reader some less common terms in medical terminology, sometimes designations (words) that had ceased to be used in the period between the creation of the text and the time of its copying, so that they had been generally forgotten.

The reverse of the papyrus, on the other hand, contains eight magical incantations (against air contaminated by infection, fever, mental breakdown, a swallowed fly, and diseases caused by demons) for the need of the physician or patient and five instructions for various cases (menstrual problems, cosmetic faults, and an inflammation of hemorrhoids), which must have been copied from another model.

It is clear that the Edwin Smith Papyrus, like other preserved medical papyri (David 2008, 186–93), is an invaluable source for research on the ancient physician's treatment of injuries and wounds based on a rational attitude.

In contrast to Smith's highly specialized text, the Ebers Papyrus (fig. 10) offers a much broader range of medical problems. It is the most extensive medical text known from ancient Egypt, and according to the indication in one of the cases (856a), the book was found under the feet of Anubis's statue in Khem (Letopolis in Greek) at the time of the reign of Den (First Dynasty), which supposedly added to its importance.

The cases from the Ebers Papyrus include diverse medical topics, covered by coherent groups of cases. The last such group, at the very end of the text (Cases 862–877), is somewhat close to the cases from the Edwin Smith Papyrus and recommends a surgical approach—"knife or glowing stick"—for the treatment of tumors, cysts, inflammations, hernias, hematomas, and ascites. The cases from the Ebers Papyrus are thus a valuable parallel to the Edwin Smith Papyrus, which deals with the area of healing in relation to injuries and other diseases: one group of cases in the Ebers Papyrus is similar in general subject to the Edwin Smith Papyrus but differs in some details and in the manner of treatment.

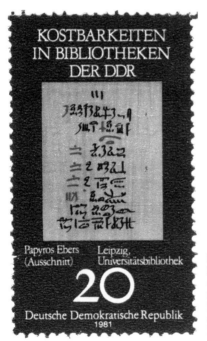

Fig. 10. In 1981, the Ebers Papyrus, the most extensive ancient Egyptian medical text, became the only one to be the subject of a postage stamp for the former German Democratic Republic.

The Ingredients of the Remedies for Surgical Treatment

The methods for treatment of injuries and other problems in the area of surgery comprised the application of remedies that were to relieve the patient's pain, speed healing, or prevent infections. The recommended curative mixtures included herbal, animal, and mineral ingredients.

We can precisely determine a number of such ingredients and judge their possible curative effect, but the importance of many others remains unknown. In such cases, we place a phonetic transcription of the Egyptian name of the substance in the text.

Neither in the cases of the Edwin Smith Papyrus nor in the selected cases of the Ebers Papyrus are the precise amounts of the remedies listed.

The ingredients of mineral origin

A raw mineral frequently used in treatment of wounds and injuries was alum *(imeru)*, which has astringent effects and is used to this day to stop bleeding from scratches or after insect bites. Bandages with alum undoubtedly had a positive effect on injuries. Natron *(netjeryt, hesmen)* is better known in connection with mummification for drying the soft tissues of the dead body, but it must also have been beneficial in medicine or healing for its absorptive or osmotic effect, helping reduce swelling. Sea salt, labeled in the texts as salt from the Delta *(hemat mehtet)*, worked in the same way.

The other useful remedies that we find in connection with specific injuries included a malachite powder *(wadju)*, which thanks to its copper admixtures helped prevent the growth of some bacteria, but it is not certain whether the Egyptians were aware of malachite's anti-inflammatory effect or whether they used it rather for its green color, symbolizing resurrection and rebirth. They also used a popular eye make-up, galenite *(mesdemet)*, verdigris *(djabet net bia)*, or cuttlebone *(nes-sh)*, a source of natural calcium and phosphorus, sometimes in ground form as a calcium powder *(deku shes)* as well. The ingredients mentioned also include stoneworker's mortar *(deben ikedu)*, which could be lime or gypsum, pumice *(weshbet)*, an igneous, porous mineral related to glass just like pulverized faience *(tjehenet)*, vitreous matter from which jewelry, decorations, or small statues were usually made. We also find among the ingredients threshing-floor dust *(seky en khin)*, whose medicinal effect is quite doubtful. What is unknown is a mineral called in Egyptian *kesenty*. We can also find it in many other branches of medicine, including women's medicine (see chapter 4). Last but not least, the production of medicines utilized pure water *(mu)*.

The ingredients of herbal origin

In the remedies recommended for the treatment of infected wounds, a whole range of herbal ingredients was used. These included leaves of various woody species, such as catclaw acacia *(shendjet)*, which has astringent effects, the sycamore fig tree *(nehet)*, cedar *(ash)*, or willow *(tjeret)*. Willow leaves help against fever and bleeding, but it seems that in antiquity the strongly antiseptic effects of the willow bark were known. Likewise in the case of other types of trees, it was possible to use not only leaves but also bark, for example with the acacia, or other parts of the plants, such as *tepau*, which may be the seeds (?) of the sycamore fig fruit. Some preparations also comprise the leaves of the *ima* tree, which is still unknown to us.

The ingredients of the medicinal mixtures further included barley *(sekhet)*, wheat flour *(deku en sut)*, and earth almonds or the tubers of edible nutsedge *(wah)*. What is uncertain is the determination of the Egyptian term *djaret*, which is sometimes interpreted as the colocynth, but it was more likely the pulp of the pods of the carob tree, which is also known as St. John's Bread. It works as a lubricant and a demulcent.

Flatulence was treated with cumin *(tepnen)*, which could endow the medicinal mixtures with a pleasant taste.

The fruits that appear as an ingredient of the medicines in surgical cases include *ziziphus jujuba (nebes)*, whose fruits have a calming and diuretic effect (increasing the excretion of water) and are also used to this day in traditional Chinese medicine. On the other hand, figs *(dabu)*, the fruits of the common fig tree, have a laxative effect. Poppy seeds *(shepnen)* had a great importance particularly as an intoxicating and stimulating analgesic. Beans or long beans *(iveryt)* were also used, and linen seeds *(desher)* and dried fiber *(fetet shu)* were beneficial as well. Unknown to us are the fruits called in Egyptian *amau* and the plant *heny-ta*, sometimes considered a variety of papyrus sedge.

The ingredients of animal origin

The most frequently used remedies in surgical treatment recommended in the cases of the Smith Papyrus included fresh (raw) meat *(iuf wadj)* and honey *(bit)*. The meat was placed on the wound during the first day of treatment to support the coagulation of the blood. Honey applied to open wounds was very beneficial thanks to its anti-inflammatory and osmotic effect, aiding against swelling.

Another frequent ingredient for treatment was oil of animal origin *(merhet)*. Animal fat *(adj)* was also used; sometimes specifically the fat of ibex, for example, was required. Milk fat *(mehwy)* was another beneficial ingredient, whereas in the more magical sphere we can include dung *(benef)*, sometimes specifically of the cow. Ostrich eggs were to help in the treatment of a fractured skull. The category of magical ingredients of the so-called *Dreckapotheke* (filth pharmacy) includes, for example, fly droppings *(hesu afef)* or dried (fly's?) blood *(senef seshu)*.

Translation of the Surgical Cases

Editorial note: Round brackets ( ) mark contemporary additions for better comprehension of the text. Square brackets [ ] mark restorations of the text that were present originally but have not been preserved. The words that appear in red ink on the papyri are set in bold type in this edition, emphasizing the important passages of the text.

Edwin Smith Papyrus
Case Smith 1: 1,1–1,12

[Instructions on the wound suffered on the (patient's) head which reaches all the way to the bone of his skull and is not opening.

When you examine someone who has] a wound on the head whose edges [are closed] and are not opening, [. . . , then you say of him: "A person with a wound] on the head. A disease that I will treat."

You must the (very) first day wrap him with fresh meat and then every day you will use bandages with oil [and honey] until he feels better.

Concerning "when you examine someone," [it refers to] an examination of someone, [similar to] a check-up using a grain measure, [like when] something [is measured] with a gauge or inspected using fingers [. . .]. Concerning a measurement of something by a grain measure [. . .], look at the impairment in the same way. Determining someone's handicap [. . . Concerning the] heart, the veins lead to it from (all) limbs. [When thus] Sekhmet's priest and physician places his hands or fingers [on the head, or on the crown] of the head, on (whichever) hand, on the heart area, or on (whichever) leg, (then) he measures (directly) the heart, because its arteries are in the crown of the head and in the heart area and because (it beats) in every artery of every limb. The measurement reveals . . . [the pulse of the heart] on the arteries of his head, the top of his head, and his feet. [The physician measures the pulse] of the heart to know what is coming out of it, because the measurement reveals to him what is happening inside.

Concerning a "wound suffered [. . .]," it means that it is a small wound, [it is not wide] and neither one nor the other (of its) edges is opening.

Concerning one "which reaches all the way to [the bone of his skull and is not] opening," it means that the flesh was cut, so that the [wound reaches all the way] to the bone of the (patient's) skull, but [neither edge] is opening, (the wound) is small and is not wide.

Case Smith 2: 1,12–1,18

Instructions on [a gaping] wound [on (the patient's) head] which reaches all the way to the bone.

When you examine someone who has [a gaping wound on the head] which reaches all the way to the bone, you must (first) place a hand on him and examine [the wound] by touch. When you discover that the skull is [intact] and unbroken, then you say of him: "A person with a gaping wound on the head. A disease that I will treat."

You must [the (very) first day wrap him with fresh meat, place two linen bands on the wound, and then] every day [use bandages with oil and honey] until he feels better.

Concerning "a [gaping] wound [on the (patient's) head which reaches all the way to the bone," it means . . .] his injury.

Concerning the "two linen bands," [they are] two [linen] bands [which are placed across the edges of the gaping wound to pull one side to] the other.

Concerning "unsplit or undisturbed," [it means . . .].

Case Smith 3: 1,18–2,2

[Instructions on] a gaping wound on the (patient's) head that reaches all the way to the bone and has penetrated [his skull.

When you examine someone who has a gaping wound on the head] which reaches all the way to the bone and has fractured his skull, you must (firstly) examine the wound by touch. When you determine that [he cannot look at his arms] or chest and that he suffers from neck stiffness, **then you say of him: "A person [with a gaping wound on the head which reaches all the way to the bone and has penetrated] his skull. A disease that I will treat."**

Once you [join] his wound [with sutures, you must apply] the (very) first day fresh [meat]. You must not bandage him. He must (remain) lying [on a bed until his illness passes].

Then you must use bandages with oil and honey every day until he feels better.

[Concerning a "gaping wound on the (patient's) head which reaches all the way to the bone and has penetrated] his skull," it is a small fracture, because (this) caused penetration is reminiscent of the cracking of a cooking pot . . .

Concerning "he cannot look at his arms or chest," [it means that for him it is not easy to look at] his arms and neither is it easy for him to look at his chest.

Concerning "he suffers from neck stiffness," it means stiffness after a previous injury which has crossed to his neck, so that the neck was thus affected.

Concerning "he must (remain) lying **on a stretcher**," it is **placing him on a stretcher** and observing him without giving any medicine.

Case Smith 4: 2,2–2,11

Instructions on a gaping wound on the (patient's) head which reaches all the way to the bone and has split his skull.

When you examine someone who has a gaping wound on the head which reaches all the way to the bone and has split his skull, you must (firstly) examine the wound by touch. When you find in it something uneven under your fingers and the (patient) has severe pains, the swelling on (the wound) is rising, the (patient) is bleeding from the nostrils and ears and suffers from neck stiffness, so that he cannot look at his shoulders or his chest, **then you say of him: "A person with a gaping wound on the head which reaches all the way to the bone and has split his skull. He is bleeding from the nostrils and ears and suffers from neck stiffness, so that he cannot look at his shoulders or his chest. A disease that I will contend with."** When you discover that the skull of that person is split, you must not bandage him. He must (remain) lying on a bed until his illness passes. The treatment is (first) in a seated (position). He will have two brick rests prepared until you know that a reversal has occurred. (Then) put oil on his head and apply it also on his neck and shoulders. In precisely this way, you deal with everyone whom you discover to have a split skull.

Concerning **"split skull,"** one skull bone is separated from the other while the bone fragments are caught in the tissue of the scalp and are not separated.

Concerning **"the swelling on the (wound) is rising,"** it means that the swelling on that split place is rising up.

Concerning **"until you know that a reversal has occurred,"** it means that you can tell whether (the patient) will die or live. Therefore, it is a "disease that I will contend with."

Case Smith 5: 2,11–2,17

Instructions on a gaping wound on the (patient's) head which has split his skull.

When you examine someone who has a gaping wound on the head which reaches all the way to the bone and has split his skull, you must (firstly) examine the wound by touch. When you discover that the split of the (patient's) skull is deep and sunken under your fingers, it has great swelling and (the patient) is bleeding from the nostrils and ears and suffers from neck stiffness, so that he cannot look at his shoulders or his chest, **then you say of him: "A person with a gaping wound on the head which reaches all the way to the bone and has split his skull. He suffers from neck stiffness. A disease that nothing can be done about."**

You must not bandage him. He must (remain) lying on a bed until his illness passes.

Concerning "split skull," it is a cracked skull when the bones of the split have fallen inside the (patient's) skull. The treatise "Dealing with Wounds" says of it: it is a shattering of the skull into many chips, fallen into the skull.

Case Smith 6: 2,17–3,1

Instructions on a gaping wound on the (patient's) head which reaches all the way to the bone, has split his skull, and exposed the brain.

When you examine someone who has a gaping wound on the head which reaches all the way to the bone, has split his skull, and exposed the brain, you (firstly) have to examine the wound by touch. When you find that the crack of the (patient's) skull has (the form of) wavy grains, like those that occur when heating copper, something is throbbing there and trembling under your fingers, like the soft spot on the crown of an infant's head before it hardens—and that the throbbing and trembling take place under your fingers because the brain in its cranium is damaged—(the patient) is bleeding from the nostrils and suffers from neck stiffness, (then it is) a disease that nothing can be done about.

You must apply oil **to his wound.** You must not bandage him. You must not place bandages on his wound until you know that a reversal has occurred.

Concerning "which has split his skull and exposed the brain," it is a large crack open to the inside of his skull (all the way) to the membrane which covers the brain, (so that) it runs from inside the skull through the crack.

Concerning the "(form of) wavy grains, like those that occur when heating copper," it is copper from which the metalworker—before pouring it into a cup—removes the impurities on the surface and which (is reminiscent) of small bumps. Like when one says "a grain of pus."

Case Smith 7: 3,2–4,4

Instructions on a gaping wound on the (patient's) head which reaches all the way to the bone and has penetrated his frontal sinus.

[When you examine someone who has a gaping wound on the head which reaches all the way to the bone and has penetrated his frontal sinus], you have to examine the wound by touch (first). When (the patient) has severe pains, make him raise his face even though it is hard for him to open his mouth and his heart weakens when he wants to speak. When you notice that saliva stays in his mouth and does not drip on the ground, that he is bleeding from the nostrils and ears and suffers from neck stiffness, so that he cannot look at his shoulders or his chest, **then you say of him: "A person with a gaping wound on the head which reaches all the way to the bone and has penetrated his frontal sinus. The muscle of his (lower) jaw has contracted, he is bleeding from the nostrils and ears and suffers from neck stiffness. A disease that I will contend with."**

When you discover that the muscle of the (lower) jaw of that person is contracted, you must put something warm on him until he feels better. He opens the mouth and you bandage him, (then you use) oil and honey until you know that a reversal has occurred.

However, when you discover that the person has a fever from the wound that is in his frontal sinus and that his teeth hurt from the wound, place a hand on him. When you find that his forehead is wet with sweat, the muscles on his neck are engorged, his face is red, his teeth and back (hurt), the box of his head smells like sheep and goat urine, his mouth is clenched, his forehead is wrinkled, and his face looks as if he were crying, **then you say of him: "A person with a gaping wound on the head which reaches all the way to the bone and has penetrated his frontal sinus. His teeth hurt, his mouth is clenched, and he suffers from neck stiffness. A disease that nothing can be done about."**

However, when you discover that the man has turned pale when he manifested weakness before, you must make a wooden peg for him, wrap it in cloth, and put it in his mouth. And have a drink from tubers of edible nutsedge prepared for him. The treatment is in a seated (position) between two brick rests until you know that a reversal has occurred.

Concerning "penetrated (his) frontal (sinus)," it is what is between two skull bones. The frontal (sinus) is as if of leather.

Concerning **"the muscle of the (lower) jaw of that person is contracted," it is the stiffening (caused) by the muscles at the end of the ramus (lower jaw)—which is attached to the temporal bone—so that (the jaw) cannot move one way or the other. For (the patient), it is not easy to open his mouth because of his injury.**

Concerning **"the muscle of the (lower) jaw,"** they are the muscles connecting the ends of his jaw, as when you tie something with a string.

Concerning **"his forehead is wet with sweat," it means that his head is** a bit sweaty, as when something is damp.

Concerning that "the muscles on his neck are swollen," it means that the muscles on his neck are swollen and stiffened as a result of the injury.

Concerning "red face," it means that the color of his face is red like the color of red fruits.

Concerning "the box of his head smells like sheep and goat urine," it means that his forehead smells like sheep and goat urine.

Concerning "box of his head," it is the center of the forehead with respect to the brain that resembles a box.

Concerning "his mouth is clenched, his forehead is wrinkled, and his face looks as if he were crying," it means that he does not open his mouth to speak, his forehead is contracted and rises and drops like the forehead of someone who narrows the eyes when crying.

Concerning "the man has turned pale when he manifested weakness before," it is turning pale in danger—as when a person encounters a poisonous snake—the result of weakness.

Case Smith 8: 4,5–4,18

Instructions on a fractured skull under the skin of the head.

When you examine someone who has a broken skull under the skin of the head and nothing is (visible) on the surface, you must (firstly) examine the wound by touch. When you find puffed-out swelling above a fracture that is in the (patient's) skull, when because of that he squints on the side on which the skull is fractured, and when walking he drags the leg on the side on which the skull is fractured, you know that he has been stricken by something from the outside; the humeral head is not free (in movement), he cannot touch the palm of his hand with his fingernail, he is bleeding from the nostrils and ears and suffers from neck stiffness. A disease that nothing can be done about.

The treatment is (first) in a seated position until he feels better and until you know that a reversal has occurred. **When you find that the crack of the (patient's) skull has (the form of) wavy grains, like those that occur when heating copper, something is throbbing there and trembling under your fingers, like the soft spot on the crown of an infant's head before it hardens—and that the throbbing and trembling take place under your fingers because the brain in its cranium is damaged—(the patient) is bleeding from the nostrils and suffers from neck stiffness, (then it is) a disease that nothing can be done about.**

Concerning "a fractured skull under the skin of the head on which no wound is (visible)," it is a fracture of his skull bone, with the surface of the head being undamaged.

Concerning "when walking he drags the leg," it concerns walking with a limp leg, which is not easy for (the patient). (The leg) is weak and staggers, the toes are turned toward the instep, and when walking they seek the ground. It means that the (patient) shuffles because of it.

Concerning "he has been struck by something from the outside" on the side where the wound is, it is the penetration by something from the outside into the side where the wound is.

Concerning "something from the outside," it is the breath of a god from the outside or the dead who appears; nothing that would be caused by the (patient's) body.

Concerning "the humeral head is not free (in movement), he cannot touch the palm of his hand with his fingernail," it refers to the fact that the humeral head is immobile, and that the fingernail cannot touch the palm of his hand.

Case Smith 9: 4,19–5,5

Instructions on an injury of the (patient's) forehead that has fractured the skull.

When you examine someone who has an injury on the forehead that has fractured the skull, you must prepare an ostrich egg smeared with oil for him and place it on the edge of his wound. Then, you must prepare an ostrich egg mashed and ground into powder for him. That is what dries the wound. Then you must apply to it a bandage from a physician's kit. You must remove it the third day and you will find that it has joined the wound, now having the color of an ostrich egg.

What is recited as a magic (incantation) over this medicine is: "The enemy who was in the wound has been cast out! The conspiracy that was in the blood has been suppressed! The usurpers of Horus who were on all sides (have ended) in the mouth of the Beneficent Goddess (= Isis)! This temporal (bone) will not be affected! There is no crocodile or poison in it! Because I am under the protection of the Beneficent Goddess (= Isis): the son of Osiris has been saved!"

Then you cool figs, oil, and honey for him. You boil it for him, cool it, and give it to him. Concerning "a bandage from a physician's kit," it is a linen band like that used by an embalmer. (The physician) must apply it on the medicine that is on the wound on the (patient's) forehead.

Case Smith 10: 5,5–5,9

Instructions on an injury that is on the (patient's) eyebrows.

When you examine someone who has a wound on the eyebrows that reaches all the way to the bone, you must examine the wound by touch (first) and (then) suture the detached part with thread. **Then you say of him: "The wound is on his eyebrows. A disease that I will treat."**

Once you have sutured it, (you must apply immediately) the first day fresh meat. When you find that the sutures of the wound are loose, you must pull them with two linen strips. You will treat his wound every day with oil and honey until he feels better.

Concerning "two linen strips," they are two linen bands. They are put across the edges of the gaping wound to pull one side to the other.

Instructions on a fracture in the pillar of the (patient's) nose.

When you examine someone who has a fracture of the bridge of the nose, such that his nose is flat, the face even, and the swelling on it puffy, and (the patient) is bleeding from both nostrils, **then you say of him: "A person with a fracture in the pillar of the nose. A disease that I will treat."**

You must clean (his nose) with two linen rolls and insert two linen rolls soaked in oil in the nasal cavities. Then you place him on a bed until the swelling goes down. You must attach two solid linen cylinders to prevent the nose from moving. Then you will apply oil and honey every day until he feels better.

Concerning "the pillar of the (patient's) nose," it is the ridge and side part of the nose and the center of the nose between the nostrils.

Concerning "the (patient's) nostrils," they are the two lateral parts of the nose passing into the cheeks beginning at the end of the nose and rising to the peak of the nose.

Instructions on a fracture in the (patient's) nasal cavity.

When you examine someone who has a fracture in the nasal cavity and you find that the nose is crooked, the face flat, and the swelling on it puffy, **then you say of him: "A person with a fracture in the nasal cavity. A disease that I will treat."**

Put the nose back in the right position. Clean the nasal cavities with two linen bands until all the blood clots dried inside the nasal cavities are removed. Then you must push two linen rolls soaked in oil into his nasal cavities. You must attach two solid linen cylinders and bandage that. You will apply oil and honey every day until he feels better.

Concerning "a fracture in the (patient's) nasal cavity," it is the center of his nose, all the way where it ends between the eyebrows.

Concerning "the (patient's) nose is crooked, the face flat," it means that his nose is askew and all very swollen, just like the cheeks, so that the face is deformed and does not have its normal appearance, because all the cavities have been affected by swelling, and the face thus looks deformed.

Concerning "all the blood clots dried inside the nasal cavities," it is a blood clot inside of the patient's nasal cavities resembling a worm living in water.

Case Smith 13: 6,3–6,7
Instructions on a fracture of the (patient's) nose.

When you examine someone who has a nose fracture, you must put your hand on his nose at the place of that fracture. When it is trembling under your fingers and (the patient) is also bleeding from the nostril and ear close to that fracture, can hardly open his mouth, and is apathetic, **then you say of him: "A person with a nose fracture. A disease that nothing can be done about."**

Case Smith 14: 6,7–6,14
Instructions on the wound in the (patient's) nose.

When you examine someone who has a wound in the nose, which is blocked, and discover that the edges of the wound are opening, you must join his wound with sutures. **Then you say of him: "A person with a wound in his nose, which is blocked. A disease that I will treat."** You will prepare two linen rolls and wipe all the blood clots dried inside the nostril. You must wrap his (wound) the (very) first day with fresh meat. Once the sutures are loose, after you have removed the fresh meat from it, you must bandage him every day (using) oil and honey until he feels better.

Concerning the "wound in his nose, which is blocked," it means that **the edges of his wound are droopy, open to the inside of the nose,** with the drooping causing the blockage.

Case Smith 15: 6,14–6,17
Instructions on a piercing of (the patient's) cheek.

When you examine someone whose cheek has been pierced and find that the swelling on his cheek is puffy, black, and strange, **then you say of him: "A person with a pierced cheek. A disease that I will treat."**

You must wrap his (wound) (using) alum, and then you will treat his wound with oil and honey every day until he feels better.

Instructions on a slash to (the patient's) cheek.

When you examine someone whose cheek has been slashed and find puffy swelling and red (coloration) around that rupture, **then you say of him: "A person with a slashed cheek. A disease that I will treat."**

You must wrap (the wound) the (very) first day with fresh meat. The treatment is in a seated (position) until the swelling goes down. Then you will treat his wound with oil and honey every day until he feels better.

Case Smith 17: 7,1–7,7

Instructions on a fracture in the (patient's) cheek.

When you examine someone who has a fracture in his cheek, you must put your hand on his face in the place of that fracture. When it is trembling under your fingers and (the patient) is bleeding from the nostril and ear on the side where the wound is and is also bleeding from his mouth and only barely opens his mouth, **then you say of him: "A person with a fracture in his cheek. A disease that nothing can be done about."** You must wrap (the wound) the (very) first day with fresh meat. Make him sit until the swelling goes down. Then you will treat his wound with oil and honey every day until he feels better.

Case Smith 18: 7,7–7,14

Instructions on the wound on the (patient's) temple.

When you examine someone who has a wound on his temple that is not gaping, although it reaches all the way to the bone, you have to (firstly) examine the wound by touch. When you discover that his temple is intact, without a rupture, piercing, or fracture, **then you say of him: "A person with a wound on his temple. A disease that I will treat."**

You must wrap (the wound) the (very) first day with fresh meat and then treat (his wound) with oil and honey every day until he feels better.

Concerning the "wound that is not gaping, although it reaches all the way to the bone," it means that the wound that reaches all the way to the bone is small and there is no rupture. This is a narrow wound, without (gaping) edges.

Concerning "his temple," it is what is **between** the end of his eye canthus and the auricle on top of his lower jaw.

Case Smith 19: 7,14–7,22

Instructions on a piercing of the (patient's) temple.

When you examine someone who has a pierced temple with a wound still on it, you must (first) examine the wound. And you will tell him: "Look at your shoulders!" If it is difficult for him, he turns his neck only slightly, and his eye on the side with the wound is bloodshot, **then you say of him: "A person with a pierced temple. He suffers from neck stiffness. A disease that I will treat."**

You must place him on a bed until his disease has passed and treat (the wound) every day with oil and honey until he feels better.

Concerning "his eye is bloodshot," it means that his eye's color is red, like the color of the anacyclus (plant). The treatise "The Skill of an Embalmer" says of it that his eyes are red and sore, as (when) the eye (is) very tired.

Case Smith 20: 7,22–8,5

Instructions on the wound on the (patient's) temple that reaches all the way to the bone and has penetrated his temple.

When you examine someone who has a wound on his temple that reaches all the way to the bone and has penetrated his temple, (whose) eyes are both blood-shot, and who is slightly bleeding from his nostrils, when you put your fingers on the opening of (his) wound, it is very painful for him, and when you ask him what is troubling him, he does not answer, tears are pouring from his eyes, and he often lifts his hand toward his face to wipe his eyes with the back of his hand, as children do without being aware of doing it, **then you say of him: "A person with a wound on his temple that reaches all the way to the bone and has penetrated his temple. He is bleeding from the nostrils, suffers from neck stiffness, and is apathetic. A disease that nothing can be done about."**

As the person is apathetic, **you must place him in a seated position, apply oil on his head, and pour rancid milk fat into his ears.**

Case Smith 21: 8,6–8,9

Instructions on the split of the (patient's) temple.

When you examine someone who has a split temple and find puffy swelling around the rupture, (the patient) is bleeding from the nostril and ear on the side where the rupture is, and hardly hears you speaking, **then you say of him: "A person with a split temple. He is bleeding from a nostril and ear as a result of that injury. A disease that I will contend with."**

You must leave him lying on a bed until you know that a reversal has occurred.

Case Smith 22: 8,9–8,17

Instructions on the crush of the (patient's) temple.

When you examine someone who has a crushed temple, you must put a finger on his chin and (another) of your fingers at the end of his ramus (of the lower jaw). He will be bleeding from his nostrils and ears as a result of that crush. You must clean the (wound) with a linen roll, and (then) you will see (bone) fragments in his ears. When you address him, he will be apathetic and will not speak. **Then you say of him: "A person with a crushed temple who is bleeding from his nostrils and ears, is apathetic, and suffers from neck stiffness. A disease that nothing can be done about."**

Concerning "the end of his ramus (lower jaw)," it is the end of his lower jaw. The lower jaw is inserted into the temple like the claw of the plover bird when holding something.

Concerning "you will see (bone) fragments in his ears," it means that bone fragments will emerge that have stuck on the roll inserted to clean the inside of the ears.

Concerning "is apathetic," it means that he does not say anything at all, is in low spirits, and cannot speak, like the one who is stunned by something that has come from the outside.

Case Smith 23: 8,18–8,22
Instructions on an injury of the (patient's) ear.

When you examine someone who has a wound on the ear that reaches all the way to the orifice while part of the auricle remains inside, you must attach it with a suture beyond the ear cavity. **Then you say of him: "A person with a wound on the ear that reaches all the way to the orifice. A disease that I will treat."**

When you find that the suture on the wound is loose but it is still holding the edges of the wound, you must prepare linen rolls for him and put them on the ear from behind. Then you will treat his wound with oil and honey every day until he feels better.

Case Smith 24: 8,22–9,2
Instructions on a fracture of the (patient's lower) jaw.

When you examine someone who has a broken lower jaw, you must put your hand on (the wound). When you find that the fracture is trembling under your fingers, **then you say of him: "A person with a broken (lower) jaw. The wound has risen but is not draining. As a consequence, (the patient) has a fever. A disease that nothing can be done about."**

Case Smith 25: 9,2–9,6
Instructions on the dislocation of the (patient's lower) jaw.

When you examine someone who has a dislocated (lower) jaw and find that his mouth is open and he cannot close it, you must insert your thumbs under the end of the ramus of the lower jaw inside his mouth and your index fingers under his chin. Then you push them (= the rami) into their place. **Then you say of him: "A person with a dislocated (lower) jaw. A disease that I will treat."**

You must wrap the wound every day with (a bandage with) alum and honey until he feels better.

Case Smith 26: 9,6–9,13

Instructions on the wound in the (patient's) lip.

When you examine someone who has a wound in the lip that reaches all the way to the oral cavity, you must (first) examine his wound all the way to the nasal septum and (then) join it with sutures. **Then you say of him: "A person with a wound in his lip that reaches all the way to the oral cavity. A disease that I will treat."**

Once you suture (his wound), you must wrap it the (very) first day with fresh meat. Then you will treat (his wound) with oil and honey until he feels better.

Concerning the "wound in his lip that reaches all the way to the oral cavity," it means that the edges of his wound are sagging and open inside the mouth. The sagginess is connected with clogging.

Case Smith 27: 9,13–9,18

Instructions on a gaping wound on the (patient's) chin.

When you examine someone who has a gaping wound on the chin that reaches all the way to the bone, you have to examine the wound by touch (first). When you discover that the bone has remained undamaged and there is no rupture or crack in it, **then you say of him: "A person with a gaping wound on the chin that reaches all the way to the bone. A disease that I will treat."**

You must apply two linen bands to the wound. The (very) first day, you wrap him with fresh meat and then every day you treat the wound with oil and honey until he feels better.

Case Smith 28: 9,18–10,3

Instructions on the wound in the (patient's) throat.

When you examine someone who has a gaping wound in the throat that reaches all the way to the esophagus, so that when he drinks water, he chokes and the (water) comes out of the hole of his wound, the wound is inflamed, and (the patient) has a fever from it, you must join that wound with a suture. **Then** you say of him: "A person with a wound in the throat that reaches all the way to the esophagus. A disease that I will contend with." You must wrap his (wound) the (very) first day with fresh meat and then every day treat it with oil and honey until he feels better. When, however, you find that he still has a fever from the wound, you put dry fiber on the opening of the wound. And he must remain lying on a bed until he feels better.

Case Smith 29: 10,3–10,8

Instructions on a gaping wound on the (patient's) cervical vertebra.

When you examine someone who has a gaping wound on a cervical vertebra that reaches all the way to the bone and has penetrated his cervical vertebra, and when you examine the wound by touch and (the patient) is in great pain and cannot look at his shoulders or his chest, **then you say of him: "A person with a wound in the neck that reaches all the way to the bone and has penetrated his cervical vertebra. (The patient) suffers from neck stiffness. A disease that I will contend with."**

You must wrap his (wound) the (very) first day with fresh meat. Then you place him on a bed until his disease has passed.

Case Smith 30: 10,8–10,12

Instructions on a tear of the vertebral (ligament) in the (patient's) neck.

When you examine someone who has a torn vertebral (ligament) in the neck, and you tell him to look at his shoulders and his chest, and he does so, but it is difficult for him to look in this way, **then you say of him: "A person with a torn vertebral (ligament) in the neck. A disease that I will treat."**

You must (immediately) wrap (the wound) the first day with fresh meat. Then you will treat it every day with alum and honey until he feels better.

Concerning "a tear," it refers to a separation of two members while (both) remain in (their) place.

Case Smith 31: 10,12–10,22

Instructions on a dislocation of the (patient's) cervical vertebra.

When you examine someone who has a dislocated cervical vertebra and find that as a consequence of this he does not feel his arms or legs, that as a consequence of this his penis is erect while urine is dripping from it without his being aware of this, that he is suffering from flatulence and his eyes are bloodshot, then it is a shift of a cervical vertebra, which has affected his spine, causing him not to feel his arms or legs. When a cervical vertebra is dislocated, it results in an erection of the penis. **Then you say of him: "A person**

with a dislocated cervical vertebra who does not feel his legs or arms and who is dripping urine. A disease that nothing can be done about."

Concerning "a dislocation of a cervical vertebra," it refers to a separation of one cervical vertebra from another while the flesh on them has remained intact, as when we say of something that should join two things but (in fact) separates them that it is dislocated.

Concerning "as a consequence of this his penis is erect," (it means that) his penis is constantly erect and has semen at its end. This means that it is upright; it does not drop or rise.

Concerning "who is dripping urine," it means that urine is constantly dripping from his penis and he cannot retain it.

Case Smith 32: 11,1–11,9

Instructions on a displacement of the (patient's) cervical vertebra.

When you examine someone who has a displaced cervical vertebra, and his face is immobile and he cannot turn his neck, and you tell him to look at his chest and shoulders and he will not be able to turn his face to look at his chest and shoulders, (then you say of him:) "A person with a displaced cervical vertebra. A disease that I will treat."

You must wrap (the wound) the (very) first day with fresh meat. Once you unbind the bandages, you use oil so that it gets to his neck. Then you wrap him (with a bandage with) alum and treat him every day with honey. And he must remain seated until he feels better.

Concerning the "displacement of his cervical vertebra," it refers to the slippage of the cervical (vertebra) to the inside of his throat, as when a foot sinks into (soggy) soil. It is sinking down.

Case Smith 33: 11,9–11,17

Instructions on a crushing of the (patient's) cervical vertebra.

When you examine someone who has a crushed cervical vertebra, and you find that one of his vertebrae has sunk into another, (the patient) is apathetic and cannot speak—while his fall on his head has caused one of his vertebrae to wedge into another—and further, you find that as a consequence of this he cannot feel his arms or legs, then you say of him: "A person with a crushed cervical vertebra who cannot feel his arms or feet and is apathetic. A disease that nothing can be done about."

Concerning the "crushing of a cervical vertebra," it refers to the wedging of one of the cervical vertebrae into another, when one falls into another without their being able to move one way or the other.

Concerning "his fall on his head has caused one of his vertebrae to wedge into another," it means that (the patient) fell on his head, and one of his cervical vertebrae penetrated another.

Case Smith 34: 11,17–12,2

Instructions on the dislocation of the (patient's) collarbone.

When you examine someone who has a dislocated collarbone and find that his shoulders are dropped while the head of his collarbone is closer to his face, then you say of him: "A person with a dislocated collarbone. A disease that I will treat."

You push it so that it sinks back into its place. You must wrap it with firm linen cylinders and then treat it every day with oil and honey until he feels better, but **when you find that the (patient's) collarbone is broken and its crack heads inward, (then you also say:) "A disease that I will treat."**

Concerning the "dislocation of his collarbone," it means that the ends of his collarbones are twisted so that the heads rest in the upper bone of his chest and protrude all the way to his throat, with the flesh around the collarbone being in place. It is the flesh that is in (the front part of) the neck, under which there are two arteries, one on the right and one on the left in the area of the neck: they (both) supply (blood) to his lungs.

Case Smith 35: 12,3–12,8

Instructions on a fracture of the (patient's) collarbone.

When you examine someone who has a broken collarbone and find that his collarbone is shortened and diverted from its other part, **then you say of him:** "A person with a broken collarbone. A disease that I will treat."

You place (the patient) on something rolled between his shoulder blades. You must spread his shoulders to stretch his collarbone and make the fracture sink back into place. You prepare two linen cushions and then place one of them on the inner side (of the upper part) of his arm and the other on the underside of his arm. **You must wrap it (with a bandage with) alum and then you treat it every day with honey until he feels better.**

Case Smith 36: 12,8–12,14

Instructions on a fracture of the (patient's) arm.

When you examine someone who has a broken arm and find that his arm hangs freely and deviates from its other part, **then you say of him: "A person with a broken arm. A disease that I will treat."**

You place (the patient) on something rolled between his shoulder blades.

You must spread his arms to stretch them and make the fracture slip back in its place. You prepare two small linen cushions for him and then place one of them on the inner side of his arm and the other on the underside of his arm. You must wrap it with (a bandage with) alum and then you will treat it every day with honey until he feels better.

Case Smith 37: 12,14–12,21

Instructions on a fracture of the (patient's) arm and a wound on it.

When you examine someone who has a broken arm and a wound inflicted on it (as well), and find that the fracture is trembling under your fingers, **then you say of him: "A person with a broken arm and a wound inflicted on it. A disease that I will contend with."**

You prepare two small linen cushions. You must wrap it with (a bandage with) alum and treat it with oil and honey until you know that a reversal has occurred. **When, however, you find that blood is flowing from the wound where the fracture is and coming from the inside, then you say of him: "A person with a broken arm and a wound inflicted on it. A disease that nothing can be done about."**

Case Smith 38: 12,21–13,2

Instructions on a fracture of the (patient's) humerus.

When you examine someone who has a fractured humerus and find puffy swelling above that fracture that is on the (patient's) arm, **then you say of him: "A person with a fractured humerus. A disease that I will treat."**

You must wrap it with (a bandage with) alum and then you will treat it every day with honey until he feels better.

Case Smith 39: 13,3–13,12

Instructions on a rash with flat-topped lesions on the (patient's) chest.
When you examine someone who has a rash with flat-topped lesions on his chest and find that it is swollen with pus, forms a (continuous) surface, and is hot when you touch it with your hand, **then you say of him "A person with a rash with flat-topped lesions on his chest that excretes pus. A disease that I will treat with a fire-drill."**

You must singe him (with a fire-drill) on his chest, on the rash that he has on his chest, and (then) treat him the way you treat wounds. Do not prevent the (rash lesions) from opening on their own; that would not be good for his disease. Every wound on his chest will be singed as soon as it opens on its own.

Concerning "a rash with flat-topped lesions on his chest," it means that the (rash) is swollen and spread all over the chest as a consequence of his disease, and has formed pus and redness on his chest. It means that it resembles something scratched up that forms pus.

Case Smith 40: 13,12–13,17
Instructions on a wound on the (patient's) chest.
When you examine someone who has a wound on his chest that reaches all the way to the bone and has penetrated his sternum, and when you touch his sternum with your fingers, it causes him great pain, **then you say of him: "A person with a wound on his chest that reaches all the way to the bone and has penetrated his sternum. A disease that I will treat."**
You must wrap the wound the (very) first day with fresh meat and then every day you will treat it with oil and honey until he feels better.
Concerning "his sternum," (it is) the upper part of his chest resembling a hedgehog.

Case Smith 41: 13,18–14,16
Instructions on an infected wound on the (patient's) chest.
When you examine someone who has an infected wound on his chest, the wound is inflamed, a hot flush is radiating onto your hand from the opening of the wound, the edges of the wound are reddish and that person has a fever from it, his flesh will not stand a compress and (new) skin is not forming on the wound, with the surface of the opening of that wound being watery and feverish and the drops coming out of it being limpid, **then you say of him: "A person with an infected wound on his chest that is inflamed and from which he has a fever. A disease that I will treat."**
You must make for him a cooling preparation that will draw the heat out of the opening of the wound: willow and ziziphus leaves and the *kesenty* mineral, **apply them on it.** (Or) the leaves of the *ima* tree, dung, *heny-ta*, and the *kesenty* mineral, **apply them on it.** You must make for him a preparation that will desiccate the wound: malachite powder, pumice, faience, and fat, **spread and wrap it.** (Or) salt from the Delta and ibex fat, **pulverize and wrap it. You must (also) prepare for him a powder** from poppy and linen seeds, cuttlebone, the carob tree, and sycamore leaves, **spread and wrap it.** If any limb is affected in any such way, you will follow the same procedure.
Concerning "an infected wound on the chest that is inflamed," it means that the wound that is on his chest is still open, does not close, hotness comes out of it, its edges are red, and its opening is open. The treatise "Dealing with

Wounds" says of it: it means that it is still very swollen; the high temperature is called inflammation.

Concerning "a hot flush in his wound," it means that the hotness affects the entire inside of the wound.

Concerning "its edges are reddish," it means that its edges are red like the color of red ochre.

Concerning "his flesh will not stand a compress," it means that his flesh will not accept the medicine because of the fever on his chest.

Concerning "a hot flush is radiating onto your hand from the opening of the wound," (it means) that the hotness from the opening of the wound is radiating toward your hand, as it is said of something that comes out and sinks that (it) returns.

Case Smith 42: 14,16–14,22

Instructions on the bruising of the ribs in the (patient's) chest.

When you examine someone who suffers from (the pain) of the ribs in his chest without there having been any dislocation or fracture, but that person suffers from great pain, **then you say of him: "A person with bruised ribs in his chest. A disease that I will treat."**

You must wrap him with (a bandage with) alum and then every day you will treat him with honey until he feels better.

Concerning "the ribs in his chest," they are the bones in his chest that are sharp, like a protruding thorn.

Case Smith 43: 14,22–15,6

Instructions on a dislocation of the ribs in the (patient's) chest.

When you examine someone who has dislocated ribs in his chest and find that the ribs of his chest are protruding and their heads are reddish and that the person suffers from swelling on both sides, **then you say of him: "A person with dislocated ribs in his chest. A disease that I will treat."**

You must wrap him with (a bandage with) alum and then you will treat him every day with honey until he feels better.

Concerning "dislocated ribs in the (patient's) chest," it is a release of the rib heads, which permanently rest in his chest.

Concerning "suffers from swelling on both sides," it means that he suffers as a consequence of their displacement in his chest, so that there is swelling on both sides.

Concerning "both sides," they are his loins.

Case Smith 44: 15,6–15,9

Instructions on the fracture of ribs in the (patient's) chest.

When you examine someone who has fractured ribs in his chest, and the fracture has a wound on the surface (as well), and you find that the ribs on his chest are trembling under your fingers, **then you say of him: "A person with fractured ribs in his chest and a fracture (that also has) a wound on the surface. A disease that nothing can be done about."**

Case Smith 45: 15,9–15,19

Instructions on round ulcers on the (patient's) chest. When you examine someone who has round ulcers on his chest and find that they have spread all over the chest, and when you put your hand on the chest on those ulcers and find that they are very cold and they are not hot at all, you do not feel anything granular, (the ulcers) are not watery, nor do they form water drops, but you have something round in your hand, **then you say of him: "A person with round ulcers. A disease that I will contend with."**

Nothing else. When you discover round ulcers on any human limb, treat them according to these instructions.

Concerning "round ulcers on his chest," it means that (the patient) has on his chest large, spread, and hard swellings that upon touch (remind you of) a stuffed ball, resembling the green husk of the trigonella, hard and cold under your hand, just like when one touches that swelling on his chest.

Case Smith 46: 15,20–16,16

Instructions on a bulging blister on the (patient's) chest.

When you examine someone who has a bulging blister on the chest, and further on (the chest) you discover a spread rash, watery under your hand, something that is sticky, but the tops (of the blisters) have not turned red, **then you say of him: "A person with a bulging blister on the chest. A disease that I will treat** with a cooling compress (applied) on the blister on his chest."

Barley, natron, and the *kesenty* mineral, **spread and wrap it.** (Or) calcium powder, the *kesenty* mineral, mortar, and water, **spread and wrap it.** If it resists these cooling measures, then you abandon this method until (in the end) all the water in the blister has come out.

Treat him like you treat wounds, thus with a preparation driving out the hotness from the opening of the wound on the chest: with acacia leaves, sycamore leaves, water, the *ima*-tree leaves, cattle dung, and the *heny-ta* plant, **wrap it. Then you will make a preparation for his chest:** malachite powder, the carob tree, cedar (leaves), fat, oil, salt from the Delta, and ibex fat, **wrap**

it. Then you prepare a compression for him: poppy, linen, and sycamore seeds, **spread them and apply them on it.**

Concerning **"a bulging blister on the chest,"** it means that on his wounded chest there is great swelling, clear like the fluid under your hand.

Concerning **"something that is sticky,"** it means that the skin is not hot.

Concerning **"have not turned red,"** it means that there is nothing red there.

Case Smith 47: 16,16–17,15

Instructions on a gaping wound on the (patient's) shoulder.

When you examine someone who has a gaping wound on the shoulder, the flesh is missing, the edges are separated, and (the patient) suffers from shoulder dehydration, **you must** (first examine) the wound (by touch). If you discover an open rupture, detached on both sides, reminiscent of an unrolled linen roll, and (the patient) can lift his arm (only) with difficulty, then you suture that rupture. **Then you say of him: "A person with a gaping wound on his shoulder, the flesh is gone, the edges are separated, and (the patient) suffers from shoulder dehydration. A disease that I will treat."**

You must wrap him the (very) first day with fresh meat. When you discover an open wound and loose sutures, pull the rupture with linen strips and then treat him with oil and honey every day until he feels better.

When you discover a wound whose flesh is missing, and the edges are separated from any human limb, you must follow these instructions.

When you, however, discover a wound, and the flesh is hot on the shoulder wound, and that wound is inflamed and open and the stitches are loose, then put your hand on it. And when (your hand) feels the hotness coming out of the opening of the wound and also water drops, as cold as raisins, **then you say of him: "A person with a gaping wound on the shoulder that is inflamed and from which he has a fever. A disease that I will contend with."**

And when you discover that the person has a fever and his wound is inflamed, you must not bandage him. He must (remain) lying on a bed until his illness passes. And once the fever has dropped and his wound is no longer hot, you must then treat him every day with oil and honey until he feels better.

Case Smith 48: 17,15–17,19

Instructions on the bruising of the (patient's) thoracic vertebra.

When you examine (someone who) has a bruised thoracic vertebra, you will tell him: "Straighten your legs and bend them!" He will straighten them, and then he will immediately bend them again, because it causes him pain because of the affected thoracic vertebra. **Then you say of him: "A person with a bruised thoracic vertebra. A disease that I will treat."** You must lay him stretched on his back. You will prepare for him . . .

Ebers Papyrus
Case Ebers 862: 105,16–106,2
Instructions on swelling (containing) pathogenic substances that has lasted (already) for many days.

When you judge swelling (containing) pathogenic substances that has lasted (already) for many days, in which pollutants and fat have formed, which is bulging and (the patient) has a fever,

then you say of it: "(A person) with swelling (containing) pathogenic substances in which pus has accumulated and pollutants have formed and (the patient) has a fever. A disease that I will contend with."

You must prepare a remedy for removing the causes: make a powder of dried blood, Roman cumin, oil, the carob tree, the leaf of the acacia tree, seeds (?) (fruit of the sycamore), the bark (?) of the acacia tree, cuttlebone, and verdigris.

Case Ebers 863: 106,2–106,7
Instructions on a tumor from the flesh on any place of the human body.

When you judge a tumor from the flesh on any part of the human body and find that it is like skin on (all of the patient's) body, (the tumor) is tight, it does not move under your fingers, it will not yield to the pressure of your fingers, and something is happening in it, **then you say of it:** "It is a tumor from flesh. A disease that I will heal with fire after examination (of the tumor)."

You will treat him like someone with whom a burning joss stick is used.

Case Ebers 864: 106,7–106,13
Instructions on a tumor at the top of the (patient's) abdomen.

When you judge a tumor at the top of the (patient's) abdomen above the navel, you must place a finger on it, feel his belly, and knead (it) with your fingers. When you make (the patient) cough, the (tumor) as a consequence of his cough rises (further).

Then you say of it: "It is a tumor on the abdomen. A disease that I will treat." It is heat in the urinary bladder in the belly that causes (the disease). And even when it (sometimes) reduces, it returns again. You must heat (the tumor) to close its path to the abdomen. You will treat him like someone with whom a burning joss stick is used.

Case Ebers 865: 106,13–106,17

Instructions on a tumor on the lower side of the (patient's) abdomen.

When you judge this (tumor) on the lower side of the (patient's) abdomen, and water rises and drops in the stomach, **then you say of it:** "The supply of air is insufficient on the lower side of the (patient's) stomach. A disease that I will treat."

It is heat in the urinary bladder in the stomach that causes (the disease). You must put a burning joss stick on (the tumor), but it must not penetrate the peritoneum. You will treat (the patient) like someone with whom a burning joss stick is used.

Case Ebers 866: 106,17–107,1

Instructions on a vascular tumor of cedar oil.

When you judge a vascular tumor of cedar oil—(where) it has been formed by (a vessel) on the abdomen (of the patient)—you feel it and it is (hard) like stone to the touch, **then you say of it:** "It is a vascular tumor. A disease that I will treat with (the aid of) a knife."

You must apply a bandage with (beef) fat on it. You will treat (it) just like wounds on any place of the (patient's) body.

Case Ebers 867: 107,1–107,5

Instructions on a fat tumor.

When you judge a fat tumor on any place of the patient's body and find that it moves away under your fingers and returns, and that it separates in parts under the (pressure of your) hand, **then you say of it:** "It is a fat tumor. A disease that I will treat."

You must treat it with (the aid of a) knife just like (another clean) wound.

Case Ebers 868: 107,5–107,9

Instructions on a tumor with the (characteristics of a) son.

When you judge a tumor with the (characteristics of a) son on any place of the patient's body and find that it is one or (there are) more, it is like skin on the (patient's whole) body, it is solid under your fingers, (but) not too much, and is large and burning, **then you say of it:** "It is a tumor with the (characteristics of a) son. A disease that I will treat."

You must treat it with (the aid of) a knife just like a wound on any place of the human body.

Case Ebers 869: 107,9–107,14

Instructions on a pus tumor.

When you judge a pus tumor on any part of the patient's body and find that its peak is raised, delimited, and globular, **then you say of it:** "It is a tumor (filled) with pus that has poured into the body. A disease that I will treat with (the aid of) a knife."

In (the tumor), there are substances similar to herbal slime, which come out of it like wax. They form pockets, and when (the remnants of) the substance remain in the pockets, they return.

Case Ebers 870: 107,14–107,16

Instructions on a tumor in the hair.

When you judge a tumor in the hair and find that it is globular and soft (but) that its content is hard, **(then you say of it: "It is a tumor in the hair.)** A disease that I will treat with (the aid of) a knife."

It looks like a tumor with pus (or) a pathogenous substance.

Case Ebers 871: 107,16–108,3

Instructions on a tumor (filled) with painful substances.

When you judge a tumor (filled) with painful substances on the (upper) ends of the arms and find that water has come out of it, and that it is solid under your fingers, immobile, and soft, (but) not too much, **then you say of it:** "It is a tumor (filled) with painful substances on the (upper) ends of the arms. A disease that I will treat." **You must treat it** with (the aid of) a knife. Be careful of the blood vessel! The substances that have come out of (the tumor) are like a water (solution) of rubber. When a pocket is around (the tumor), you must not allow the (remnants of) the substances to remain in it, (because) the (tumor) could return. You must treat it just like a wound on any place of the human body. (Once) it closes and (the state of) the blood vessel improves, (the place) may after the removal (of the tumor) become swollen. The germs of the painful substances can harm the patient.

Case Ebers 872: 108,3–108,9

Instructions on a vascular tumor.

When you judge a vascular tumor on any place of the human body and find that it is globular and hard under the pressure of your fingers, separated from the (surrounding) flesh (of the patient), it does not enlarge and does not form a peak, **then you say of it:** "It is a vascular tumor. A disease that I will treat." It is caused by blood cells. (The tumor) can also change into a vascular injury. **You must treat** it with (the aid of) a knife heated in a fire. (Then, the tumor) does not bleed too much. You will treat him like someone with whom a burning joss stick is used.

Case Ebers 873: 108,9–108,17
Instructions on a vascular tumor.

When you judge a vascular tumor on the inner layers (of the skin) on any place of the human body, the fact that the (tumor) is solid is clear to you (already) by looking at it, and (the tumor) is not twisted, (the blood vessels) have formed numerous knots, and (the tumor) looks like something that is blown up with air, **then you say of it:** "It is a vascular tumor."

You must not place a hand on (the tumor), (because) this is an injury of the body on the place (of a blood vessel). **You must** improve the (state of the) blood vessels on all of the (affected) areas of the patient's body.

What should be said as a real magical incantation for (the tumor): "May you flow, you vascular girdle, holding me braided and jumping between these parts of (my) body! May you not join the society of Khonsu!"

When you judge Khonsu's tumor, (you should recite the magical incantation): "You who lead (Ra), who is pleasant, protect me (too)! May you allow me to submit to Ra the Leader (Maat), Shining, at the sunrise!"

Recite four times early in the morning.

Case Ebers 874: 108,17–109,2
Instructions on Khonsu's tumor.

When you judge Khonsu's tumor, which is large and is on any place of the human body, it is uneven, has created numerous (other) tumors, something has emerged with (the patient) as if there were air in it, the tumor causes injury—and as in the previous (case) you must enchant—(but) it is not like those (numerous) tumors, (because) it endeavors to smooth out (itself) and form a scar, and every part of the (patient's) body where it appears is under pressure, **then you say of it:** "It is Khonsu's tumor." Do not do anything to it!

Case Ebers 875: 109,2–109,11
Instructions on tumors on any place of the human body.

When you judge the tumor of tumors on any place of the human body, you must (first) place a bandage on it, and when you discover that (the tumor) leaves and returns (under your fingers) and sticks to the flesh that is under it, **then you say of it:** "It is an appearance of tumors."

You must treat it with (the aid of) a knife, where the (tumor) is cut in half by a flint knife and grasped with tweezers, (hence) the tweezers must catch what is inside. Then you must cut it out with a flint knife. If there is (only) one thing reminiscent of a mouse stomach (?) inside, you must cut it out with a knife without reaching the delimitation on the edges (of the tumor) and touching the flesh. To be held in a flask of any colocynth. (The tumor) that is (as large) as a head is (treated) the same way.

Case Ebers 876: 109,11–109,18
Instructions on (a vascular tumor) of cedar oil on any place of the (human) body.

When you judge a vascular (tumor) of cedar oil on any place of the body and find that it has turned red and is arched like a bump caused by the stroke of a staff (or) the blow of some object on whatever place of the body, and (the blood vessel) has formed seven knots, **then you say of it:** "It is a vascular (tumor) of cedar oil."

You must treat it with (the aid of) a knife, (hence) a rush adapted (to the form of a surgical) knife. When the (tumor) is large and bleeding, you must burn it with fire. You will treat him like someone with whom a burning joss stick is used.

When (however) you find (it) on the inner layers (of the skin) on any place of the body, coiled like a snake and inflated with air, (then you say of it): "It is the enemy of the blood vessel."

You may not place a hand on such a thing, because it is a fatal case.

Case Ebers 877: 109,18–110,9
Instructions on the swelling of Khonsu's bloodshed.

When you judge the swelling of Khonsu's bloodshed on any place of the human body and find that it has a pointed peak and even bottom, the eyes (of the patient) are green and inflamed, and his body is therefore hot, be careful, (because) it is (the result of magical) incantation.

Also when you find (swelling) on both shoulders (of the patient), arms, groins, and thighs, and there is pus in it, do not do anything with it!

When, however, you find that it resembles any kind of swelling on the wound (or) bruising and (is located) on the chest, nipples, (or) any (other) place on the body, the (swelling) leaves, returns, and caves in under your fingers, and on the outside water forms (on it), **then you say of him:** "It is in (my) hands."

You must prepare for the (patient) medicine for quenching (swelling). Mix fly droppings, wheat flour, natron, threshing-floor dust (?), beans, galenite, and oil with the fruit *amau*, without adding water. Administer the medicine (until the time the patient) is well.

Surgical Treatment of Injuries and Other Illnesses
Injuries of the cranial vault
Smith 1 and 2

The first two cases of the Smith Papyrus discuss a wound in the soft tissues (of the scalp or galea aponeurotica, comprised of skin, subcutis, and a thin layer of muscle tissue) reaching to the surface (periosteum) of the skull cap (calvaria). In the first—lesser—case, it was most frequently a slice wound that was not open; in the second—more serious—a stab or blunt gaping wound. With the first, inspection by the physician seems to have sufficed during the examination; with the second, the physician had to use touch (palpation) to verify the character of the wound and primarily whether it may have caused a fracture of the skull bone. If not, he could in both cases announce a favorable forecast (prognosis), expressed by the decision "A disease that I will treat."

In treating a visually clean, non-festering, and recent wound, it was necessary the first day to place on it the meat of a freshly slaughtered animal, held with a linen bandage. Meat was understood as muscle tissue that is richly supplied with blood and thus containing biological agents (vitamins, hormones, and antibodies), which could favorably influence the healing of the wound. The meat usually came from small animals (sheep, goat) from the domestic herds common in rural areas and in towns. In Egypt, linen bandages were considered the ritually and materially cleanest cloth, so that they were used not only in medicine but also in the mummification of the dead.

With the gaping wound described in the second case, it was recommended to apply two linen bands on the edges of the wound, which pulled them together, instead of the more demanding suturing of the wound. In the next days, the healing of the wound was accelerated by the application of a bandage impregnated with a mixture of heated oil and honey. In Egypt, oil was one of the most diverse types of basic medical, cosmetic, and hygienic preparations. As for honey, modern experiments have confirmed its antibiotic characteristics (Estes 1989, 68–71), which could favorably influence the healing of wounds. Treatment with meat, with oil and honey, sometimes with the addition of alum (potassium phosphate) acting on the tissue as an astringent, is also repeated in a number of other cases, so that we list it in other commentaries as "standard." The use of honey was recommended in thirty of the forty-eight total cases of the Smith Papyrus (Hofmann 2008, 41–42).

The explanatory notes (glosses) in the first case that start with the words "Concerning . . ." clarify the idea of the examination or inspection of the patient. That is compared to the accuracy of measurement using a gauge, a wooden vessel for determining the amount of grain. It also included the palpation of the wound with the fingers, as the glosses also mention.

In another explanatory note, the author of the papyrus or whoever copied it accurately explains the examination of the pulse and the connection between the pulse and the heartbeat. According to the text, the pulse was examined by physicians and also the priests of Sekhmet, the goddess of illness and health, who served in her temples. The text at the same time shows that physicians already knew, entirely correctly, that from the heart, the driving force of the organism and simultaneously the center of a number of its most important functions, there lead tubes (blood vessels) to all of the limbs, in which the heart "speaks." The physician then was able to find and measure the pulse, most likely by comparison with his own pulse, and thus reveal—if he was healthy himself—an acceleration or deceleration of the patient's pulse. He recognized in this way "what is happening inside (the organism)" and thus managed to assess the patient's overall condition.

Smith 3

This case deals with a more severe wound to the head with neurological consequences. A gaping wound to the scalp that had fractured the patient's skull bone could have been caused by the sharp impact of a pointed weapon (knife, dagger, arrow) or the blow of a hammer. On the edges of such a wound, bone fragments occurred, which could be depressed into the meningeal layers of the brain, and fractures of the surrounding bone radiated in all directions from the edges of the defect (Brawarski 2001, 14). The note describes it as a small injury, reminiscent of the cracking of a cooking pot, so that its treatment had a favorable prognosis, but it caused stiffening of the patient's neck, which did not allow him to turn his head to look "at his chest or arms." The stiffening of the neck muscles in this case was most likely caused by irritation of the brain's wrappings (meninges), specifically by their bleeding (hematoma), rather than by their infection (meningitis). It was, however, necessary to place the patient on a bed and examine the wound in the standard way, as in the two previous cases.

Smith 4

A much more severe case of a gaping wound on the head with a fracture of the skull bone could be caused by an axe or an edged weapon. According to the first note, some of the fragments were caught in the tissue of the scalp. The physician had to feel (palpate) the wound, where he felt the bumpy surface of the chips from the edges of the bone defect. The patient complained of severe pains and chills; swelling rose around the wound from the bleeding (subgaleal hematoma). The severity of the injury was revealed by bleeding from the nose and ears, which signaled damage to the front and central segments of the base of the skull. The neck stiffness was a consequence of the meningeal irritation, as in the previous case (Brawarski 2001, 16–20). The twice-mentioned rising of the swelling reveals that the blow was strong, connected with a cerebral concussion (commotion). The chill came from a fever or from cramps (Pahl 1985–86, 112). The severity of the case is reflected in the uncertain prognosis: "A disease that I will contend with."

In the treatment, it was explicitly forbidden to wrap the wound (let alone suture it). The patient was to be led to a quiet place, preferably seated, supported in his armpits by two low walls built for that purpose from unfired brick according to the height of his figure. This tense position was to alternate with stretching on a bed to rest. This was to be done until a reversal occurred—a critical moment decisive of life or death. Smearing the head, neck, and shoulders with oil could only alleviate the unbearable pain (palliative care). An analogous case is mentioned by Pahl (1985–86, 112) (fig. 11).

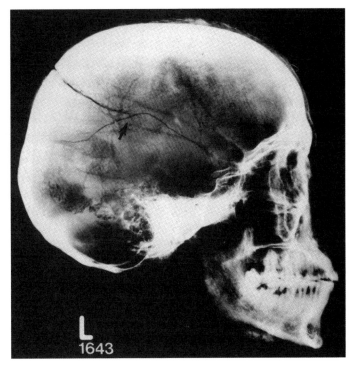

Fig. 11. Injury of the cranium reminiscent of Case 4 of the Edwin Smith medical papyrus. (After Pahl 1985–86, p. 112, Abb. 22)

Smith 5

A very severe case mentions, besides a gaping wound of the scalp, a fragmented (comminuted), sunken, or compressed (depressed) fracture of the skull bone. Its anatomical structure is reminiscent of a sandwich: it has an internal and external solid (compact) table, between which there is a soft, spongy bone (diploë). Through palpation, the physician was to determine the extent and depth of the fracture. Whereas in the previous two cases, there was a fracture of only the outer solid layer and kneading of the trabeculae of the diploë, in this case the inner bone table has also been broken as a consequence of the violent injury. It arises from the gloss that the fragments of the broken bone fell all the way to the inside of the cranial cavity, which is filled with the brain, protected by three layers of wrappings. The patient had the same, more severe symptoms as in the previous case. The prognosis was therefore inauspicious: "A disease that nothing can be done about." According to the instructions, the wound was not to be wrapped; it was necessary to place the patient on a bed and wait to see if his injury would heal itself after all. A similar but healed case was discovered by Pahl (1985–86, 125) (fig. 12).

Smith 6

This is the most severe case of a gaping wound on the head, with fragmented fracture of the skull, tearing of the meninges, and uncovering of the surface of the brain itself, which (according to the note) bends out from inside the skull. During palpation, it is possible to find in the opening of the skull wrinkling similar

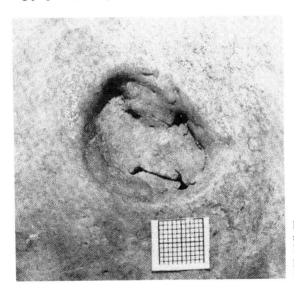

Fig. 12. A healing injury similar to Case 5 of the Edwin Smith medical papyrus. (After Pahl 1985–86, p. 125, Abb. 31)

to that which emerges from impurities in the melting of copper in the slag, which is trembling and throbbing. It is similar to feeling an infant's pulse in the area of the anterior fontanelle where the coronary and sagittal planes meet.

The other symptoms are the same as with both the previous cases, and the prognosis is similarly inauspicious. In spite of that, even in this hopeless case the author recommends smearing the wound with oil to alleviate the patient's pain and—if an unanticipated reversal of the illness occurs—wrapping it.

In the first note, the author reveals his knowledge of the membrane that covers the brain. It is evidently the thickest, and thus the most easily distinguishable, layer of the three brain membranes, the hard meninx (dura mater). In the second note, he compares the undulation of the broken skull to small bumps reminiscent of the impurities on the surface of melting copper.

In most of the translations of this case according to the interpretation of Breasted and Luckhardt (Breasted 1930, 167, 173), it is stated that this is the first evidence of the knowledge of brain foliation (gyrification). This was emphatically denied by the neurosurgeon Brawarski (2001, 9), who, based on his experience as a surgeon, considers it to be impossible, since the gyrification of a prolapsed brain cannot be identified because of the swelling.

Smith 7

In the case of another gaping wound with penetration of the skull, the *tepau* was disrupted; the translation of this word has been disputable from a medical perspective for a long time (see below). Besides a thorough palpation of the defect, the physician asked the patient to lift his face despite the severe pain. He thus knew that the patient could not open his mouth, and his heart weakened when he tried to speak. This connection arises from the conception of the heart as the motor and center of diverse functions of the organism, which included also the ability to speak. Nevertheless, it is something else: the inability to spit out saliva arises from a locking of the mouth as a consequence of a cramp of the muscles of mastication (trismus). Bleeding from the nose and ears reveals a severe state with a fracture of the cranial base, and stiffening of the neck shows a meningeal irritation. In spite of that, the physician could attempt a cure. He recommended applying something warm for blood perfusion and relaxing the muscles so the patient could open his mouth. Then, the physician treated the wound in the usual way (with warm oil and honey).

Another situation arose if a wound of this type caused a high fever with irritation of the trigeminal nerve (nervus trigeminus), manifesting itself in toothache, and the nerves evoking backache. Sweat appeared on the patient's forehead and (as a consequence of a cramp) his neck musculature constricted.

The pierced forehead cavity (sinus frontalis) stank like sheep and goat urine, and the patient's mouth was clenched and his eyebrows and facial musculature wrinkled, so that it looked as if he were crying. This picture precisely corresponds to the illness "stiffening of the neck," a wound infection by the tetanus bacterium *(Clostridium tetani)*, even though there is no mention of tonic cramps (opisthotonus), during which the body of the patient can move up into an arch. It is correctly qualified as a hopeless prognosis—the patient will die of asphyxiation (acute respiratory insufficiency) as a consequence of spasticity of the breathing musculature or heart failure. Nevertheless, not even in this case are treatment instructions lacking in response. They address the manifestations of overall weakness and pallor of the patient's face. A wooden peg wrapped in cloth and placed in the mouth not only made it possible to feed mashed food to the affected person but also protected him from biting his tongue. A drink from the tubers of edible nutsedge strengthened and calmed him, because the illness took place in full consciousness. The seated position was recommended, as with the head injury in Case 4.

The first note clarifies the term *tepau*. The original translation by Breasted (1930, 185), 'squamae,' or the 'temple scales,' or generally the translation 'seams' (sutures), has been adopted by many authors, most recently Allen (2005, 77). They are serrated bone edges fitting into one another "between one skull bone and the next." But they are definitely not "as if of leather," except at a very young age, when they do not fit together yet and are connected by fibrous connective tissue. Ebbell (1939, 26) therefore doubted the sutures and proposed the tentorium cerebelli, and von Deines and Westendorf (1962, 948) the falx cerebri, both of which are intracranial brain structures lying deep in the skull and thus hardly reachable in an injury of the cranial vault (Chapman 1992, 38). The same author (1992, 40–42) pointed out that it further says in the same sentence that "It is what is between two plates of his skull," which corresponds to one of the adjacent nasal cavities. From them, only the sinus frontalis lies between the external and internal tables of the frontal bone, resembling a "box of the head." Its relatively thin walls can easily be pierced even by a weaker blow (impressed fracture). Its epithelium (membrane) could remind the papyrus's author of leather. We mention in the fifth note that the neck muscles of the injured person are swollen and stiff as a consequence of a cramp from a tetanus infection, and in the sixth that the red color of the face was caused by a high fever (usually between 39 and 40°C).

The description of the symptoms of a tetanus infection mentioned in the text can be found in every modern medical handbook. We can admire the powers of observation of the author and the fitting formulation of the clinical manifestations of the disease. It shows his logical thinking, which can correctly be considered as scientific. Nevertheless, doubts of the diagnosis of tetanus have been expressed by Brawarski (2001, 9).

Smith 8

Another case describes a fragmented and depressed fracture of a skull bone hidden under the undamaged skin of the scalp (galea aponeurotica). By palpation of the scalp, it is possible to determine bulging caused by bleeding (hematoma) or swelling on the site above the fracture.

In observing the patient, strabismus is evident on the same side, caused by a paralysis of the optic muscles or nerves at the cranial base. That is joined, again on the side of the injury, by a defect of his walking—the muscles of one of the legs are lax, so that walking is difficult, uncertain, and swaying. It involves the actual foot turning upward in a dorsal flexion and its toes "seeking the ground." In addition, the movement of the arm is limited—the humeral head in his shoulder cannot move and a volar flexion of the hand is sluggish ("touch the palm of his hand with his finger nail").

This is again a very fitting description of the paralysis of one side of the body (hemiparesis) which was caused by a blow (commotion) to the movement (motor) center of the brain. At the same time, there was a fracture of the cranial base, manifested in bleeding from the nose and ears, and a meningeal irritation, evident from neck stiffness.

What may seem curious is the author's claim, repeated three times, that hemiparesis appears on the side of the injury, because we know that the nerve paths above the level of the large occipital opening cross (chiasma), so that the paralysis must have occurred on the opposite side. Interpreters of this part usually consider contrecoup, that is, that the blunt force that broke the skull on one side caused a paralysis on the opposite side by the motor area hitting on the wall of the skull. They also concede the possibility that the author of the text or the one who copied it confused the sides. In any case, the prognosis of such an injury had to be inauspicious.

In the part on the treatment of a fracture of the skull bone hidden under the skin, we are surprised by the palpation description of the surface of the skull, which repeats the information from Case 6 as well as its inauspicious prognosis. Might it be proof of the excellent physical examination skills of an ancient Egyptian surgeon, who even through the layer of the scalp managed to recognize the waviness of the brain surface as well as its throbbing and trembling?

In the notes, the author attempts among other things to explain the emergence of the subcutaneous fracture of the skull as a consequence of the detrimental effect of the breath of a god or a dead person, even when in reality it was most likely caused by a blow from a blunt object (contusion). In any case, it is "nothing that would be caused by the body" of the injured person.

Injuries of the forehead
Smith 9
With an injury that has fractured the patient's forehead, a description of the examination is surprisingly lacking; it has been replaced by an immediate prescription of the treatment. Instead of the standard method, this is based on the use of a fresh ostrich egg mixed with oil to smear on the edges of the wound and egg mashed and ground into powder for drying the wound. Ostriches lived in Egypt as early as prehistoric times and were a popular quarry during a hunt in the desert. In the New Kingdom, particularly in the Ramesside Period (Nineteenth and Twentieth Dynasties), they were even caught live and bred in captivity (Houlihan 1996, 166–67). The physician was to wrap the wound with a bandage, and after its removal, allegedly on the third day, the bone had fused (in reality after a longer period) and attained the color of an ostrich egg. The prognosis for the case is missing; it was most likely uncertain.

Of all of the preserved contents of the Edwin Smith Papyrus, only in this case is a recitation of a magical incantation prescribed when applying the medicine; in its text, the frontal bone was evidently mistaken for the temporal bone—apparently through an error of the scribe who copied the text. The incantation refers to the ancient myth of the goddess Isis and her son Horus, whom she protected through her magical power from danger caused by the insidious god Seth. It was popular to invoke Isis's magical power and her protection in the treatment of diverse diseases, particularly in connection with births and infants (see chapter 4), especially when the physicians were unable to help the patient in any other way. Along with the incantation, which shows the severity of the injury, the text recommends a rational treatment with a fig boiled with oil and honey.

At the end of the case, a note clarifies what a bandage is and compares it to the roller bandages used by embalmers in wrapping mummies.

Smith 10
After the severe injuries described in the previous part of the text, this is a less serious wound on the eyebrows, although it reaches all the way to the bone.

After palpation, the physician was to suture it with thread. The mention of sutures appears in more cases of this papyrus, and sewing was also part of the process of mummification, when after removal of the internal organs and drying of the body, the mummification incision in the left side was closed with thread (Smith 1912). The prognosis was good, the method of treatment common, and the sutures, if loose, needed to be pulled together by sticking with two linen bands.

Injuries of the nose
Smith 11
The first three cases of the fracture of the nose are ordered by severity in the text. The first deals with the nasal septum (septum nasi), which is cartilaginous in the front, bony in the back. Along with Ebbell (1939, 33) as well as Allen (2005, 81), we tend in this least serious case toward a fracture of the cartilaginous part of the nose. This results in a flattening of the nose and face and swelling in the surrounding areas. The fracture is accompanied by bleeding from the nostrils, a consequence of the disruption of the rich vascular network in the nasal mucous membrane. Recovery is almost certain.

In the treatment, it was necessary to clean both nasal cavities with linen rolls and then press two linen tampons into them to stop the bleeding. The cure was accelerated by placing the patient on a bed. Two solid linen cylinders stabilized the nose from both sides so that it would heal properly. Oil mixed with honey was a standard accompaniment of the treatment, most likely to speed the retreat of the swelling.

Smith 12
The case of another fracture in the nasal sinus deals with the back, bony part of the nasal septum, formed below by the vomer bone, above by part of the ethmoid bone (lamina perpendicularis ossis ethmoidalis). Its fracture, accompanied by swelling, causes distortion of the nose and hence deformation of the surrounding face. It is also an injury with a good prognosis.

The broken bone fragments first needed to be returned to their proper place (repositioned) by touch. Then, both nasal cavities were cleaned of blood clots and other impurities using two linen bands. The physician subsequently pushed two tampons soaked with oil into them for an unspecified time, which stopped the bleeding. At the end, he fixed the position of the accreting bone septum with two solid linen rolls and fastened them into place by wrapping the face. Oil with honey accompanied the treatment and most likely accelerated the retreat of the swelling.

The "cavities affected by swelling" causing a flattening of the face mentioned in the second note could be the adjoining nasal cavities, as Allen states in his translation (2005, 83).

Knowledge of the process of coagulation is apparent from the third note, where it is compared to a water worm (it could be a *Campodea*; see Ebbell 1939, 34).

Smith 13

Another case of a one-sided nose fracture is unfortunately presented too briefly. Based on the palpation finding of "trembling" (crepitation), that is, movement of the bone fragments in the location of the fracture, bleeding from one of the nostrils and ear on the same side and also from the mouth, difficulty opening the mouth, and apathy (the patient's shock), it is possible to consider a comminuted fracture, complicated apparently also by a fracture of the cranial base. It did not have to be limited only to the structure of the nose, but could also affect the upper jaw, namely its nasal edge or the frontal process of the maxilla (processus frontalis). It was caused by trauma to one side. The prognosis of the injury was hopeless, so the treatment was dropped.

Smith 14

The case of a nose blocked with a blood clot from an injury is, on the other hand, favorable in prognosis. The wound gaping on the edge of the nostril, thus in the cartilaginous part of the nose, needed to be cleaned, joined by a suture, covered first with fresh meat, and then repeatedly wrapped using oil and honey.

Injuries of the cheek
Smith 15

The cases from this group deal with injuries of the face, most likely the patient's cheekbone. In this first case, the bone was pierced and the area around the wound was affected by a strange black swelling. For a favorable prognosis, the injured person was to be treated with a bandage using alum, which has astringent and disinfecting effects, and over the next days he was to be treated with the standard method. The strange black-colored swelling led Ebbell (1939, 37) to express the idea that it was a case of noma (cancrum oris), a necrotic disintegration of the facial tissues, which affects the patient in a decrepit state with lowered immunity. This, however, would not have been possible to heal successfully at that time.

Smith 16

On the other hand, a minor case of a slash wound on the cheek with red edges as a consequence of an early infection could be cured well by the standard method. The seated position was recommended until the swelling of the cheek abated.

Smith 17

A fracture of the cheekbone, which forms the base of the face, manifested itself during palpation through trembling (crepitation), which revealed its fragmented character. This was joined by warning signs on the same side of the face such as bleeding from the nostril and ear from a disruption of the cranial base and, moreover, bleeding from the mouth and the inability to open it. The patient was in shock. It is a hopeless case, although the text recommended the standard treatment in the seated position until the swelling of the cheek abated.

Injuries of the temporal bones

Smith 18

Injuries of the temporal bones are also arranged by severity. In this case, it was a small, narrow wound, which when palpated was found to have penetrated all the way to the temporal bone without breaking it. It could be cured by the standard method.

Smith 19

A case with a small perforation of the temporal bone in connection with a wound above it needed to be examined and the patient asked to turn his neck. It was difficult for him, and his eye on the side of the injury could be bloodshot (a hematoma in the white of the eye). Nevertheless, it was possible to treat the injured with the standard method, namely lying on a bed. The red color of the sclera is compared in the note to the coloration of pellitory *(Anacyclus pyrethrum)*, and the appearance of the painful and tired eye to a description in an unpreserved treatise with the interesting title "The Skill of an Embalmer."

Smith 20

In contrast, the case of the bursting of the temporal bone caused by a blunt blow from a weapon or another object is accompanied by bleeding into the eyes and from the nostrils, great pain, and neck stiffness. The patient was semiconscious, did not answer questions, cried, and automatically wiped his tears with the back of his hand. We agree with the opinion of Ebbell (1939, 44) that these were signs of a cerebral concussion (commotion). The prognosis was hopeless. In spite of that, the physician recommended seating the patient upright, wiping his head with oil, and pouring milk fat into the ears, which works as a means to alleviate pain (palliative).

Smith 21
The milder case of the split of the temporal bone with swelling and bleeding from the nostril and ear on the side of the injury, which blocks hearing, was evaluated with an indecisive prognosis. Surprisingly, the method of treatment is missing in the text; the text only recommends quietly lying on a bed until the crisis is overcome by the natural immunity of the organism.

Smith 22
The most severe of the series of cases of an injury in the temporal area was its crushing by a comminuted fracture. The examination was to determine whether the lower jaw was cracked as well, or whether it was broken close to the temporomandibular joint. Bleeding from both nostrils and the ears indicated a simultaneous fracture of the cranial base. The patient was apathetic from the concussion, apparently semiconscious, and could not speak. It was clearly a hopeless case; therefore, any kind of treatment is lacking. The first note proves the excellent observational ability of the ancient Egyptian anatomist in a description of the shape and articulation of the lower jaw. The second explains the possible presence of bone fragments in the ears, that is, external auditory meatus, if they have stuck on the roll used inside the ears for cleaning. The third explains the patient's apathy as the effect of stunning by some evil force coming from the outside.

Injuries of the ear
Smith 23
The torn injury of the auricle reached all the way to the edge of the external auditory meatus. It is a minor case in terms of prognosis, which was resolved by suturing. When a suture became loose, it was possible to support the ear from behind with linen rolls.

Injuries of the lower jaw
Smith 24
This brief case describes a fracture of the lower jaw, which was according to the "trembling under the fingers" apparently fragmented, with a raised but not festering wound. The case was evaluated as unfavorable, most likely because of a fever from blood poisoning (sepsis). The text therefore lacks a description of the treatment.

Smith 25

The setting (reposition) of a dislocated lower jaw was described very accurately. The recommended method corresponds to the classical medicine of ancient Greece (Corpus Hippocraticum) and is used to this day in modern medicine. A bandage with alum and honey had an astringent and simultaneously anti-inflammatory effect, alleviating the pain after a dislocation. The prognosis was favorable.

Injuries of the lip

Smith 26

Another case is surprising proof of the ability of the ancient Egyptian surgeon to suture a wound even on such an exposed place as the lips, which are richly perfused with blood, even though certainly not with a suture like those of today's plastic surgeons. Quick healing was to be achieved by the standard treatment. The prognosis was also favorable in this case.

Injuries of the chin

Smith 27

An accurately described and easily comprehensible examination of a gaping wound on the chin was to rule out disruption of the bone. The case had a favorable prognosis with the standard method of treatment.

Injuries of the throat

Smith 28

On the other hand, a gaping perforated wound in the throat that reached the esophagus and caused shortness of breath while drinking could be infected, so that the prognosis in this case was uncertain. The author was aware that the patient's fever was caused by an infection of the wound, but he recommended that the wound be sutured immediately, apparently to prevent the patient from suffocating to death. However, as a consequence of such a procedure, it was possible that the fever lasted, that is, the infection continued. In such a case, it was recommended that dry fiber be put into the wound, which had to be open, to serve as drainage to remove the pus (Allen 2005, 91). According to the instructions, the patient was to remain in bed until he felt better.

Injuries of the cervical vertebrae

Smith 29

Another five cases describe severe injuries of the cervical vertebrae, whose prognosis alternates from the auspicious to the inauspicious. With the first of them, a gaping wound that reaches all the way to one of the cervical verte-brae, pain and the reflex constriction of the neck musculature did not allow the patient to turn his head. The prognosis was uncertain. Standard treat-ment with a compress with meat was recommended, but a subsequent appli-cation of a bandage with oil and honey is no longer mentioned in the text; it may have been understood by itself.

Smith 30

The title of this case and its continuation can be interpreted in several ways. The Egyptian scribe speaks of "a torn vertebral ligament." It could not be the massive, continuous anterior or posterior longitudinal ligament, but only the ligament joining the arcs of two cervical vertebrae (ligamentum interar-cuale), and perhaps also the connective tissue sheath of the intervertebral joints. In that case, both vertebrae remained in place. Ebbell (1939, 50) labels the injury as a distortion, Brawarski (2004, 65–66) as a tear of the ligaments and muscles, Allen (2005, 91) as a sprain. The movement of the neck to the sides was only slightly limited. It was a short-term strain of the vertebral connection, which could be caused by a blunt blow from behind, and whose prognosis was favorable and the treatment standard.

Smith 31

In contrast to the previous case, this is a severe case of a dislocation (sub-luxation) of one of the vertebrae of the upper and middle cervical spine. The author of the papyrus does not mention whether the vertebra shifted forward (ventrally) or backward (dorsally). In both cases, the shift could cause a nar-rowing of the spinal canal (canalis vertebralis) with resultant compression or complete transection of the spinal cord (medulla), which in a patient would be manifested as "he does not feel his arms or legs." With this description, the author documented the paralysis of all of the limbs (quad-riplegia) with their simultaneous insensibility as a consequence of a disrup-tion of the motor and sensory innervation. Penile erection (priapismus) with dripping urine occurs with the overfilling of the bladder usual with a shift of a vertebra ventrally (Brawarski 2004, 69, 71). On the other hand, the emis-sion of semen, mentioned in the second note, does not belong to the image of a transverse disruption of the spinal cord, according to the same author (2004, 67, 69). Another symptom, namely that the patient "is suffering from flatulence," was explained by Ebbell (1939, 51–52) with the idea that "his flesh (that is, musculature) accepted air," adding that the Egyptians incor-rectly considered paralysis as a consequence of the penetration of air into the muscles. He based it on a mention in Case 100 of the Ebers Papyrus (Ebbell 1939, 14–16). According to Allen (2005, 91), "he has become gaseous"; Brawarski (2004, 67) considered it to be flatulence (meteorism) as another sign of a complete transverse disruption of the spinal cord. The original symptom "bloodshot eyes" was translated by Ebbell (1939, 52) as "narrow drooping of the eyelids" (ptosis), as a consequence of a lesion of the sympathetic nerves (Horner's syndrome; Brawarski 2004, 68). The prognosis of this case was understandably inauspicious, so that the text did not even mention palliative treatment.

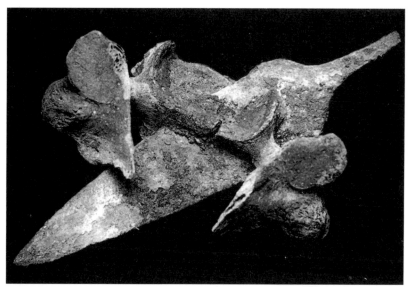

Fig. 13. A piercing of a cervical vertebra by an arrowhead that lodged in it is one of the proofs of military skirmishes in Nubia. (New Kingdom, Dakka [tomb 98.762], after Firth 1915, Pl. 38e)

Smith 32

The interpretation of this case, which describes a "shift" of a cervical vertebra, is unclear. According to the note, it was the "slippage of the cervical (vertebra) to the inside of his throat," which was compared to the sinking of a foot into (soggy) soil and dropping down. Allen (2005, 93) called this case an instruction for the setting of a displaced cervical vertebra. Ebbell (1939, 53) interpreted the dislocation as sinking to the inside of the throat downward. According to Brawarski (2004, 72), however, it was a hidden injury of the vertebra, which manifested itself on the contour of the central line of the neck with a depression (small pit) but did not cause the serious neurological symptoms described with the previous case (with the exception of the impossibility of turning the neck, perhaps because of pain, blood contusion, and swelling). He considered the case as a fracture of one or several spinal thorns (processus spinosi) created by exertion (with a single vertebra) or direct impact (with more vertebrae). With this interpretation, treatment with fresh meat does not correspond to an injury supposedly covered by skin (meat was usually placed on open wounds), just like the use of oil, alum, and honey, unless it was to have a merely psychotherapeutic effect. At the same time, the prognosis of this case was certainly good, and the text recommended that the patient remain seated until the situation improved.

Smith 33

On the other hand, the next case is severe and accurately describes the crushing (compression) of one of the cervical vertebrae by a higher-placed vertebra having fallen and wedged into it (impaction). It could happen as a consequence of a fall of the injured person headlong, directly onto the head. With the narrowing of the spinal canal by displacement or interruption of the spinal cord, there was a complete paralysis (quadriplegia) and a loss of feeling in all of the extremities. The patient was either apathetic and could not speak as a consequence of a concussion or was unconscious. The prognosis is unfavorable, and there was a danger of almost certain death, so that the text did not even provide palliative care.

A physician could not determine the diagnosis of this case visually, considering the undamaged skin. He had to rely on data on the mechanism of the injury if there was a witness, and on the patient's neurological symptoms, but it cannot be ruled out that he could recognize the change of the position of the vertebral thorns by palpation, which would prove his surprisingly high qualifications.

We have recently discovered a similar case of the incarceration of the fourth cervical vertebra into the fifth vertebra in the skeletal remains in a Ptolemaic tomb in Saqqara, in the excavations of the British Egypt Exploration Society, as well as the Dutch Museum of Antiquities and Leiden University (fig. 14). According to the solid adhesions and other reparative changes on the vertebrae, it is clear that the injured survived such a severe injury as if by miracle, although he probably remained paralyzed in all four limbs and required constant care (Strouhal and Horáčková 2007).

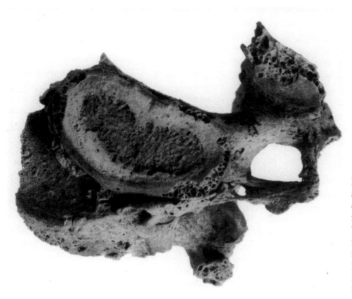

Fig. 14. The changes and adhesion after an injury are evident on the fourth and fifth cervical vertebrae. This individual survived the serious injury but remained paralyzed in all four limbs. (Ptolemaic Period, Saqqara, photo: E. Strouhal and L. Horáčková)

Injuries of the collarbones

Smith 34

The case of the dislocation of both collarbones (clavicles) had a relatively simple course with a favorable diagnosis. It occurs rarely; the dislocation is usually one-sided. The description of the examination is clear; the prognosis is expressed as auspicious twice. After repositioning the bones back into their place, it was necessary to set (fix) them with solid linen rolls and apply oil and honey to alleviate the pain.

The anatomical description in the note, however, is incorrect. It mentions the "heads" (that is, the sternal ends) of the clavicles resting in the "upper bone of his chest" (sternum), while their acromial ends should have moved all the way to his throat, with muscles ("flesh") attached to them. On both sides in the frontal part of the neck it is possible to feel two arteries (arteriae carotides), which, however, supply blood not to the lungs but to the head.

Smith 35

A broken collarbone was evident at first sight and could be successfully treated. The physician laid the patient down and placed a rolled pad between his shoulder blades. By spreading both shoulders, he achieved an extension of the clavicle, and the broken fragments slipped back into place (reposition). By placing a linen cushion on the inner side of the upper part of the arm (the humerus), and another on the underside of his flexed forearm, both fixed tightly to the trunk, he assured the maintenance of the correct position for the accreting clavicle. A bandage with alum and the application of honey eased the pain.

Injuries of the humerus
Smith 36
Not even the setting of a fracture of the humerus was a problem. The treatment was similar to the previous case; moreover, by pulling the arm the broken fragments could be repositioned. Subsequently, linen pillows were placed on both sides of the bone, serving as splints. The standard method with alum and honey ensured the success of the treatment.

Smith 37
Another fracture of the humerus in this case tore the skin, so that a wound opened above it (an open fracture). During palpation, the physician felt under his fingers the trembling of bone fragments (a comminuted fracture), so that prognosis was uncertain. The treatment was the same as in both previous cases, but if the wound caused by the fracture began to bleed (apparently complicated by infection), the prognosis changed to unfavorable.

Smith 38
The entirely minor case of a crack (infraction) of the humerus without disruption of the bone manifested itself only by swelling. According to the text, the prognosis was favorable and the standard treatment was recommended, but it is not clear from the text how the ancient physician could distinguish between a crack accompanied by swelling and swelling caused by a contusion without an x-ray.

Diseases of the chest
Smith 39
This is the case of a rash on the chest, whose blisters with a flat head (pustules, "heads") created pus, and the hands of the examiner felt heat from it. According to the note, it was a continuous swelling spreading on the patient's chest as a consequence of some illness. It created pus, almost redness, symptoms of the infection, and itched, as suggested by "something scratched up." In an explanation considering the fact that the Smith Papyrus deals with wounds, Nunn (1996, 168) deduced a secondary infection emerging from an injury, but the text itself speaks explicitly of a rash, not an injury.

The prognosis was favorable in treatment using cauterization. It is an ancient method, proved effective in North Africa from the distant past (Dastugue 1967, 1975; Strouhal and Jungwirth 1981) and in folk medicine in Nubia to this day (Strouhal 1980, 1981, 2007a). The treatment lay in scorching the painful place or a specific point on the body with the white-hot tip of a wooden or metal stick (a fire-drill). Such a method liquidates the pathological forms (for example, warts or furuncles), removes infection, or alleviates pain by a derivative effect (as with Chinese acupuncture). In our case, the rash lesions were to be left to open on their own and only then singed with a fire-drill.

Smith 40

A fitting description of a wound with perforation of the sternum, painful to the touch, which surprisingly had a good prognosis. The standard treatment was recommended. According to the note at the conclusion of the case, the shape of the upper part of the sternum, with insertions of the clavicles and ribs, reminded the author of hedgehog prickles.

Smith 41

The case graphically describes an inflamed open wound on the chest that caused a fever in the injured person and would worsen if it were bandaged. The wound had reddish edges, which the surrounding skin did not close (epithelialization) even though a clear tissue fluid (not pus) flowed from it. The prognosis for healing was, however, favorable.

According to the recommended treatment, it was necessary to cool and dry the wound. A selection of numerous herbal medicines or substances of another (mineral or animal) origin was available for that. To cool the wound, willow leaves, the leaves of ziziphus (a bush growing in semiarid areas), and an unknown mineral, *kesenty*, were used. An alternative medicine could be prepared from the leaves of an undetermined tree *ima*, dung, the *heny-ta* plant, and again the *kesenty* mineral. For drying the wound, a mixture of malachite powder, pumice stone, faience, and animal fat, which might have served as a binding agent, was useful. Another possible medication was a mixture of sea salt, which has an osmotic effect, and ibex fat. For the bandage, a mixture of poppy and linen seeds, cuttlebone, the carob tree, and sycamore leaves was prepared.

According to an explicit mention in the text, it was possible to use these recommended preparations for treating the same type of wound anywhere on the body. The first note, clarifying an inflamed wound and its main symptom, a high fever, mentions the existence of a so-far undiscovered treatise, "Dealing with Wounds." The following notes explain the features of the wound: its hot flush, its reddish edges, the inconvenience of using a compress, and the recurrent course of the fever.

Smith 42

The case of a very painful bruising (contusion) of the chest by a blunt blow had a good prognosis. The treatment with alum and later with honey to alleviate the pain was recommended. The note exaggeratedly compares the pointedness of the rib to a thorn. Perhaps that is why Ebbell (1939, 64) interpreted this case as an infraction of the ribs.

Smith 43

In another case, the situation was a dislocation (luxation) of several ribs in the sternocostal joints. Their sternal ends ("heads") stuck out under the skin and appeared reddish as a consequence of a hematoma. The injury was accompanied by swelling on both sides, which was related to the loins. We would not have expected them there, because the swelling should have been on both sides of the chest. The prognosis was good, and the treatment with alum followed by honey was recommended.

Smith 44

Another case of a fracture of the ribs is described very briefly in spite of the fact that its prognosis was inauspicious. It was an open fracture of the ribs that tore the skin above them and was trembling (crepitating) upon palpation, because the ribs had been shattered by an external trauma. The slightest attempt at treatment is lacking in the text. The physician had to be aware that the patient would die because of the certainty of infection.

Smith 45

The account of a case of round structures on the chest, which are described as ulcers or hard swellings in a note, is unique and disputable. They were spreading all over the chest, had a cool surface, their composition was not granular, and they did not contain or form any fluid. According to the note, these "swellings" were large, spread, as hard as a stuffed ball, resembling the fresh husk of the trigonella. It was a disease that the physician decided to contend with, but a recommended method of treatment is entirely lacking in the text; it might have been left out by mistake by the scribe who copied the text.

The nature of the ulcers and the cause of their emergence are not clear from the text. They were considered to be benign or malignant tumors by Ebbell (1939, 66–68). With the latter diagnosis, the prognosis would have been inauspicious.

Although no treatment is mentioned, the author of the papyrus stated that the circular structures could erupt on any part of the body and are to be "treated according to these instructions," which, however, are lacking in the text.

Smith 46

The case of a patient with a blister rising on the chest is discussed in much more depth. Its top had not turned red and, according to the first note, contained a clear fluid. It was accompanied by a watery and sticky rash. The treatment was auspicious. It lay in the application of a cooling compress of barley, natron with an osmotic effect, the unknown *kesenty* mineral, bricklayers' mortar, and water. This achieved an emptying of the content of the blister without having to pierce (puncture) it, but a wound remained that could become septic and thus had to be treated with similar medicines to cool and dry it, as in Case 41. Moreover, the leaves of the acacia and cedar were recommended. The second note in the conclusion of the case clarifies that the blister broke out on the chest in connection with an injury.

Injuries of the shoulders and back

Smith 47

The palpation examination of a gaping wound on the shoulder (above the shoulder blade) with a large defect of the tissue and detached edges, which were curled up like a roll of linen cloth, is described in detail. It was a treatable injury. When the physician, by palpation, discovered a rupture, because of which the patient could lift his arm only with difficulty, he had to suture it; if the sutures became loose, he pulled it together with linen bands. The rest of the treatment was standard.

An alternative situation with an uncertain prognosis emerged if the wound became inflamed, hot, and open, the sutures loosened, and the patient suffered a fever. He was not allowed to be bandaged so that the wound could get rid of the secretions; he had to remain recumbent, and his discomforts were lessened with oil and honey.

Smith 48

The last case, a contusion of one of the thoracic vertebrae, is not written down in its entirety. Despite the fact that free space remains on the papyrus, the scribe stopped writing in mid-sentence.

In the examination, the physician was to ask the patient to bend and then straighten his legs. In this movement, the affected vertebra was revealed by pain. The physician could treat the illness. First, he laid the patient stretched on his back, then he prepared a medication for him whose composition is, however, missing in the text.

Treatment with a Knife and Glowing Stick

At the end of the Ebers Papyrus (and also in the Hearst Papyrus, which is extracted from it), we find a series of sixteen cases considered as preserved remnants of a supposed original "Book on Tumors," where these are arched structures (bumps, bulges, protuberances, swellings) of various origin and only rarely tumors, mostly benign. They are usually labeled with the Egyptian term *aat*, singularly as *henhenet, anut,* or *shefet*. With ten of them, treatment with a knife was recommended, and with another four, treatment with a glowing stick (cauter). Since the majority of the contents of the Ebers papyrus are prescriptions on the conservative treatment of internal and other special illnesses, which will be discussed in the second and third volumes of *The Medicine of the Ancient Egyptians*, we have decided to place these sixteen cases where they belong thematically, in this chapter on ancient Egyptian surgery.

Benign tumors

Ebers 863

This case describes the treatment of a tumor that grew from the "flesh," that is, the soft tissues of the body, and that could appear on various places of the body, where, like the surrounding skin, it did not move and was tight, like leather. The prognosis was good when employing cauterization with a glowing stick. It could be a benign solid tumor emerging, for example, from connective tissue (fibroma).

Ebers 866

Another tumor is labeled a "tumor of cedar oil," formed on the abdomen of the patient. Upon palpation, it was hard, reminiscent of a stone or a lump of fat (Westendorf 1999, 704n268). It was a vascular tumor. The physician treated it with a knife and then by applying a bandage with the fat of cattle, thus like a wound on any place of the body. Nunn (1996, 167) considers that it could be a benign vascular tumor (hemangioma), even though the clinical description does not characterize it in more detail.

Ebers 867

A tumor that could form on any part of the body, that moved during palpation and was so soft that it could be separated into parts under the pressure of the hand. The treatment was auspicious. It was necessary to remove it with a knife and treat it like a clean wound. It was undoubtedly a subcutaneous benign fat tumor (lipoma).

Ebers 872

A tumor in the blood vessels on any part of the body, which during palpation appeared globular and hard, movable, and separated from the surrounding tissues of the patient. Usually, it was not large or sharp, but it had the tendency to develop into an ulcer (ulcerate). It is a treatable disease. It was operated on with a knife, which was to have been heated in a fire. The tumor did not bleed much. Then the physician was to treat it with cauterization. In this case, the diagnosis of hemangioma is much more likely (Nunn 1996, 167).

Ebers 873

Another case of a tumor of blood vessels under the skin could occur on various places of the body. It looks hard, not twisted or swollen. The blood vessels had formed many knots and the tumor appeared inflated with air. The physician was not allowed to disrupt such a structure during palpation, because a wound might appear over the vessels. Instead, he had to take care to improve the state of the vessels on all of the affected places of the body. Nevertheless, the way to do this is not mentioned in the text. Nunn (1996, 167) diagnosed this tumor as a benign blood tumor full of larger and smaller cavities (cavernous hemangioma). A surgical intervention was not recommended, evidently because of the danger of bleeding to death, so that it was necessary to resort to treatment by magical incantation, which addresses the disease itself and asks it to leave the patient's body. We can also find the same type of incantation in the treatment of women and children, for example in the collection of incantations *Book for Mother and Child* (see chapter 4).

The structure was not to develop into the so-called Khonsu's tumor (Westendorf 1999, 707n276). When the physician considered Khonsu's tumor, he was to use the magical formula: "You who lead (Ra), who is pleasant, protect me (too)! May you allow me to submit to Ra the Leader (Maat), Shining, at the sunrise!"

This magical incantation refers to Ra, the god of the Sun and ruler of the heavens, the creator of the world, whose heavenly pilgrimage symbolized perfection, government, and the constancy of the order of the world *(maat)* (for instance Assmann 1995). The *maat* order made life possible for people and the gods and was personified by the goddess Maat, depicted as a woman with an ostrich feather on her head (Wilkinson 2003, 150–52). In this incantation, she is referred to with the epithets "Leader" and "Shining," because if the patient observed the essentials of *maat*, the god was to allow his healing.

A cyst in the hair

Ebers 870

A "tumor" in the hair was globular and soft but its contents hard; on the outside, it looked like a "tumor" with pus or a substance causing diseases *(arewet)*. The treatment with a knife was auspicious. According to Nunn (1996, 167), it was a skin cavity (a dermoid or fat cyst) or a rarely occurring skin fold on the lower end of the spine (pilonidal sinus), containing hair.

Inflamed bulges

Ebers 862

Swelling *(henhenet)* is described, which had already lasted for several days and contained most likely pus and fat, and the patient had a fever. It corresponds to today's diagnosis of a small suppurative tuber (abscess), or bigger ones (furuncle or carbuncle). The prognosis was therefore uncertain. We would have expected a surgical procedure, either puncture or incision of the abscess, but instead the text recommends a mixture of several types of plants, including carminative Roman cumin, the carob tree, acacia leaves and bark with astringent effects, the seeds of the sycamore, cuttlebone, and dried blood (perhaps of flies?) dissolved in oil.

Ebers 869

A suppurative tumor that could appear anywhere on the body was an abscess, which, according to Egyptian conceptions, had originated in the soft tissues of the body. The peak of the tumor was globular, raised, and sharply defined. It contained substances similar to herbal slime, which came out of it like wax. It formed pockets in which remnants could remain, and the tumor could thus start to grow again. Treatment with a knife had a favorable prognosis.

Ebers 871

"Water" had come out of the "tumor" (more correctly, abscess) filled with a painful substance *(wekhedu)* on the upper ends of the arms. It was immobile and soft to semisoft. It could be treated with a knife, but it was necessary to be careful of the blood vessel where the fluid had been caught, which had come out of the tumor and resembled an aqueous solution of rubber (mucopurulence). If a pocket formed around the blood vessel, the physician could not allow the remnants of pus to remain in it, because the tumor could return. After the intervention, the wound could be treated like any other on any place on the body. After the removal of the tumor, the place could become swollen after healing, and germs of the painful substance could harm the patient. According to Nunn (1996, 76), this could have been abscesses of the lymphatic nodes in the armpits (axillae).

Umbilical hernia
Ebers 864
The supposed "tumor" was actually a bulge under the skin on the top of the patient's abdomen above the navel. The physician was to place his fingers on it (palpate it) and ask the patient to cough, and he saw that the bulge increased. It was undoubtedly a typical umbilical hernia, which we can also find in a number of depictions from Egyptian tombs (fig. 15). The prognosis was favorable. The treatment, however, proceeded from the incorrect opinion that the illness was influenced by heat in the region of the bladder. At the same time, the physician noticed that the hernia disappeared and constantly returned—apparently in the change of the body's position from lying to standing. It was therefore recommended to close the path of the hernia by heating it, again with a glowing stick (cauterization), which could actually harm the patient.

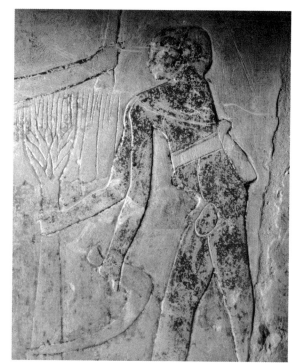

Fig. 15. Umbilical hernia can be found in the reliefs as early as the Old Kingdom; it appears particularly in the depictions of the ordinary population of the Nile Valley. (Fifth Dynasty, Mehu's tomb at Saqqara, photo: M. Zemina)

A bulge caused by subcutaneous bleeding
Ebers 876
When a physician examined another "tumor of cedar oil" (*sefet*; also see Ebers Case 866) on a blood vessel on any part of the body and discovered that it had turned red, was arched like a bump created by a blow of some object, and that the blood vessel had formed seven (meaning 'many') knots (Westendorf 1999, 708n283), he was to treat it with a knife made from a rush. If, however, the bulge was large and bleeding, it had to be burned by fire. It was then necessary to treat the patient with a glowing stick.

When, however, the physician found this structure under the inner layers of the skin, coiled like a snake and inflated with air, which was believed to fill the blood vessels along with water, he was not allowed even to place a hand on it, because it was a hopeless (fatal) case. Ebbell (1939, 127n1) expressed a diagnosis of hematoma; Nunn (1996, 168) and Westendorf (1999, 708–709) agree.

A bulge caused by a parasitic cyst
Ebers 875
In examining the "tumor of tumors" *(aat net aaut)* on any place, the physician was to place a bandage on it (according to Westendorf 1999, 707, it is an error of the scribe: correctly 'his fingers') to recognize that it was moving while being stuck to the flesh, that is, to the surrounding soft tissues. It was recommended that the "tumor" be incised with a flint knife to make it possible to grasp whatever was inside with tweezers and cut it out with a knife. If there was something in there that was reminiscent of a mouse stomach (?), the physician had to remove it with a *shas* knife, without reaching its edges and touching the surrounding tissues, and was to place it in a flask of colocynth. Even a "tumor" as large as a head was to be treated the same way. Miller (1989) believes that it was the cyst of a Guinea worm *(Dracunculus medinensis)*. The "innards of the mouse" could refer to the intestines, which most likely reminded the physician of the shape of the female of this parasite.

A bulge caused by fluid in the abdominal cavity
Ebers 865
Another supposed "tumor" arched on the lower side of the patient's abdomen, in which water rose and dropped. The physician considered the cause to be an insufficient air supply on the lower side of the abdomen. He intended to treat the disease and thought that it was influenced by an infection of the bladder. Nunn (1996, 166–67) considers the cause of the described bulge to be the effusion of tissue fluid into the peritoneal cavity (ascites). As a treatment the author recommends

piercing the abdominal wall with a knife *(hemem)*, analogously to the method that Aulus Cornelius Celsus described in the first century AD (*De medicina* VII, 15: 1). In contrast, Westendorf (1999, 704) agrees with treatment by cauterization, but the burning must not penetrate the peritoneum into the abdominal cavity.

Bulges of uncertain origin

Ebers 868

A mysterious tumor "with the characteristics of a son" (Westendorf 1999, 704n269), which Nunn (1996, 167) translates as "with the characteristics of a goose," could be found on any place of the body, namely as one or more structures. Upon palpation, they were solid but not hard, like the skin of the patient's body, large, and burning. Treatment was possible by removal of the tumors with a knife and treating the wounds left from them. According to Westendorf (1999, 704n269), it could be an eruption of daughter deposits of a destructive tumor (metastases); it has not yet been proved, however, that these were known in ancient Egypt.

Ebers 874

This case describes the appearance of a so-called Khonsu's tumor, which was large, could appear on various parts of the body, had an uneven surface, and formed many other tumors *(anut)*, perhaps metastases. It appears as if there were something filled with air inside the body of the patient. This tumor hurts the patient but at the same time attempts to smooth itself out and form a scar. Every part of the body that had such a tumor was under pressure, and the physician was not to do anything against it, except for incantation. It was thus either a tumor that had managed to heal itself—for example, a blister bursting with the departure of a worm (Bardinet 1995, 196, 371)—or on the other hand a hopeless case. Nunn (1996, 168) proposed several diagnoses: cancer (carcinoma), a dermatological form of leprosy, plague tubers (pestis bubonica), or von Recklinghausen's disease (neurofibromatosis).

Ebers 877

Swelling *(anut)* caused by "Khonsu's bloodshed," which could appear on any place on the body, was characterized by a pointed peak and even bottom. The patient's eyes were green and inflamed and his body was therefore hot, which seems to have revealed an infection. According to the conceptions of Egyptian physicians, this disease was caused by a harmful magical incantation. The physician was instructed to do nothing if swellings with pus appeared on the arms, shoulders, thighs, and groins. If, however, they appeared in the form of swelling from the wound or bruising on the chest, nipples, or in any other place of the body, and if they moved or collapsed upon palpation and water was excreted from them and was visible on the outside, it was necessary to act. The medicine administered was a mixture of a purée from wheat flour, oil, threshing-floor dust, natron, galenite, beans, the unknown fruit *amau*, and fly droppings, which was apparently to act magically.

A number of authors, beginning with Ebbell (1939, 84–85), judged it to be leprosy, for which, however, any evidence is lacking in Egypt in the dynastic period. Nunn (1996, 75, 168) states the same diagnoses as in Ebers Case 874. "Khonsu's bloodshed" refers to the ancient Pyramid Texts, where this god helped the king in slaughtering and eating the heavenly gods, which likely symbolizes the superiority of the sun and moon (king and Khonsu) over the stars (heavenly gods) (Wilkinson 2003, 113–14).

Surgeons and Their Treatments
The question of the existence of specialized surgeons

Having read the previous chapters, we may ask whether the outstanding observational and palpational abilities of the Egyptian or the rationality of their prognoses and treatment methods is the work of physicians–specialists who devoted themselves only to surgery. Among the various specialized titles of lay physicians, called *sunu* (or *sinu*), none have yet been found that would relate to operations. The question is if the hieroglyphic symbol *sun* (◀——◌) had some connection with operations (Nunn 1996, 115). Also connected with surgical operations were the priests of the temple of the goddess Sekhmet, who according to ancient Egyptian religious beliefs sent down illnesses to people but, placated by prayers and sacrifices, allegedly also healed them. Nevertheless, the evidence for this claim is inconclusive.

Other than the severe and minor injuries described in the Smith Papyrus or the tumors, cysts, and other diseases from the Ebers Papyrus, we do not have any written proof from ancient Egypt of the surgical treatment of other illnesses. The reliefs in the tombs, faithfully depicting diverse aspects of everyday life, do not capture the course of surgical operations; similarly, depiction of mummification is lacking. The reason was the holy purpose of the tomb depictions, which was to ensure the owner a safe existence in the afterlife. Since the reliefs could be magically revived, it was not desirable to include in them the negative aspects of life, like serious illnesses, injuries, or operations. The exceptions are the possible depictions of circumcision, which we know from the mastaba of Ankhmahor, the vizier and director of all the works of King Teti in Saqqara (Sixth Dynasty) (fig. 16); from the wall of the temple in

Luxor from the time of Amenhotep III (Eighteenth Dynasty); and from the temple of the god Khonsu the Child in Karnak (Twenty-second Dynasty). If it really was a circumcision, it is interesting that it was performed by temple priests and not physicians, namely with a traditional flint knife. It could be a ritual of the ceremonial acceptance of pubescent boys among adult men. The physician Spigelman (1997) believed that these scenes might capture an emergency surgical operation—the release of an inflamed and swollen glans penis. More recent studies of these depictions and particularly of the accompanying hieroglyphic legends have, however, shown that it was rather the depilation of the funerary priest around his genitalia, which was prescribed for Egyptian priests as a component of their ritual cleansing (Grunert 2002, 150; Vachala 2007a, 661). Moreover, in Ankhmahor's tomb the scene of the 'circumcision' is accompanied by a depiction of a manicure and pedicure, which would corroborate this interpretation (fig. 17). The other two above-mentioned scenes of 'circumcision' from later temples, however, have not yet undergone a similar discussion.

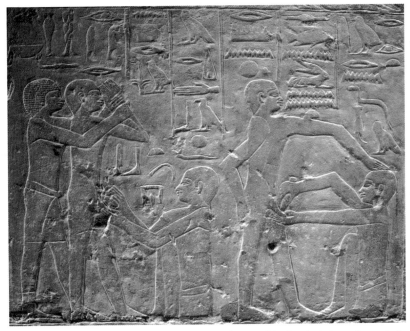

Fig. 16. The scene of a 'circumcision,' considered to be one of the few depictions of a surgical procedure in Egyptian reliefs, has recently been reinterpreted as a scene of ritual shaving. The accompanying hieroglyphic inscriptions explain that it is the scene of the 'Purification of the Burial Priest.' (Sixth Dynasty, tomb of Ankhmahor at Saqqara, photo: M. Zemina)

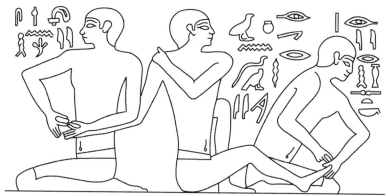

Fig. 17. Manicures and pedicures were among the customary procedures for the maintenance of hygiene in Egyptian society. (Sixth Dynasty, tomb of Khentika at Saqqara, drawing: H. Vymazalová after James 1953, Pl. XI)

The depictions of work injuries on a relief from the Deir al-Medina tomb (TT 217) of Ipui, builder of the royal tombs in the Valley of the Kings dated to the Twentieth Dynasty, are also unique. A colleague's sledge hammer has fallen on the foot of one of the stonemasons; another man, with the aid of a stick or a straw, is removing a foreign object from the eye of a colleague; and in another part of the scene a man, perhaps a physician, is resetting the dislocated right shoulder of a recumbent laborer (fig. 18).

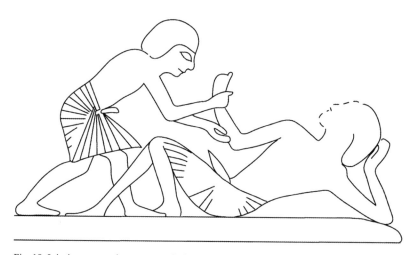

Fig. 18. Injuries seem to have occurred often, including among workers in craft workshops. This scene portrays the resetting of a dislocated shoulder. (Twentieth Dynasty, Ipui's tomb [TT 217] at Deir al-Medina, drawing: H. Vymazalová after Davies 1927, Pl. 37)

Some of the treatment methods of severe injuries described in the Smith Papyrus suggest that they proceeded from the experience of military physicians. Although there is no proof of such a specialization among the Egyptian titles either, physicians or healers accompanied military campaigns from the earliest periods and hence acquired a great deal of experience in the treatment of war injuries (traumatology). Moreover, the nature of many of the wounds mentioned in the Smith Papyrus indicates war injuries or other violent acts.

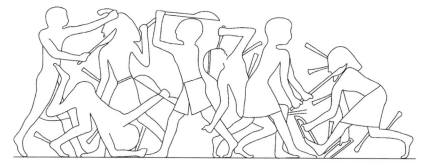

Fig. 19. Egyptian healers had to treat many slash and stab injuries during military campaigns. (Fifth Dynasty, Inti's tomb in Deshasha, drawing by H. Vymazalová after Petrie, Deshasha, Pl. X)

A study of the skeletal remains and mummies, when conducted by physicians or anthropologists with experience in paleopathology, has so far revealed only very rare evidence of surgical operations. The most famous example of a fatal war injury can be found on the head of the mummy of the penultimate king of the Seventeenth Dynasty, Seqenenre Tao. This brave king fell in battle with the Hyksos, when he was struck with five wounds on the head and face. Two of them (fig. 20) were demonstrably caused by Asiatic battle axes used by Hyksos warriors (Bietak and Strouhal 1974).

At the time of medicine's beginnings, it is not possible to expect large surgical operations inside the body; on the other hand, there were minor surgeries to cure conditions on the surface of the body. These included opening (incision) of boils (furuncles) or abscesses, treating injuries and ulcers, setting dislocations or fractures, amputations, trepanations, and other minor operations, for example, help in childbirth complications (see chapter 4). They were most likely performed by the more skillful members of the category of general lay physicians—*sunu*.

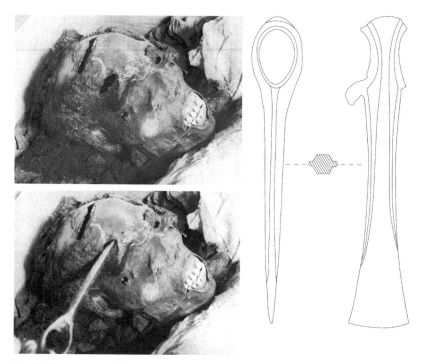

Fig. 20. The mummy of King Seqenenre displays the war injuries that he suffered in battle with the Hyksos. Of the five injuries to the head (a), two were demonstrably inflicted by a hatchet of the Middle Eastern type, such as the Hyksos war hatchets (b, c). (Seventeenth Dynasty, Egyptian Museum, Cairo [CG 61051], after Bietak and Strouhal 1974, fig. 4, tab. 3, 4)

We thus encounter the initial phase of the advancement of medicine— minor surgeries without specialized surgeons, hence a kind of protosurgery (Sullivan 1998).

Examination of the patient to determine a diagnosis and prognosis

In order for the physician to be able to examine and heal the sick properly, the student of medicine had to study for a certain time in the libraries and scriptoria called 'houses of life,' where the knowledge of various scientific branches was gradually accumulated (Strouhal 1992a–c, 235–42). By studying the medical scrolls there, preserved in cylindrical pigeon-holes in the walls of those buildings, the medical student first acquainted himself with the knowledge of anatomy and physiology, the pathophysiological concepts of health and illness, and later also diseases and instructions or recipes for curing their symptoms. Prepared in this way, he was ready to treat the sick, first perhaps accompanying an older, experienced colleague to his house, where the patients would come, or directly to the residences of the patients.

Most of the cases of the Smith Papyrus, surprise us today by the precision of the physician's visual observation and capability for fine feeling (palpation) both in the inspection of the content of an open wound and in determining the states and positions of the bones and any bone splinters in the hypodermis.

The author or authors of the papyrus seem to have created the terminology of the anatomic structures of the human body by comparing them with phenomena in nature and everyday life. So, for instance, they called the end of the ramus of the lower jaw (processus muscularis et condylaris mandibulae) "bird's claw with two fingers"; the sinus frontalis "the box of the head," "secret chamber," or "holy of holies"; and the ridge or partition of the nose (dorsum seu septum nasi) the "column of the nose." Other times, they compared the observed structures to different phenomena, such as the cracking of the skull to the cracking of a ceramic vessel or brain gyrification to the puckers of metal slag.

In another case of a fragmented fracture, they discussed the rupture of the brain meninges ("the bag covering the brain"). Whereas the physiological conception considered the brain as a mere resource and reservoir of liquids, coming out of it to the surface of the head through its "seven holy orifices" (the eyes, ears, nostrils, and mouth), the authors of the papyrus in the examination of an injured person determined that his wound affected the motor or sensory functions of other organs.

They did not connect a patient's shock, semiconsciousness, or unconsciousness with the brain, but they recognized them from experience. They knew bleeding from the nose, ears, and mouth to be a sign of a severe, hopeless status without even knowing that it was a fracture of the skull base. They also noticed the important symptom of stiffening of the neck without knowing of an irritation of the brain meninges.

They recognized another source of nerve control in the spine in cases of injured vertebrae, but they did not identify the spinal cord and understand its function. They did manage, however, to graphically express paresis and the loss of feeling of the limbs (insensitivity) by the phrase "he does not feel his arms and legs."

The determination of these important neurological symptoms relied on an examination of the motor abilities of the injured if he was conscious and able to perceive the spoken word. The physician gave him instructions to tilt his head and look at his chest, to turn his head to the side and look at his shoulders, and so on. On the other hand, we lack information on the previous course of the disease (anamnesis—medical history), perhaps because the causes were evident with injuries caused by external force.

Careful examination combined with experience led the physician of the Smith Papyrus to judge the severity of the patient's status and expression of the forecast of the further development of his disease (prognosis) on a three-stage scale: (1) "a disease that I will treat," (2) "a disease that I will contend with," (3) "a disease that nothing can be done about."

Surgical instruments and aids

In the Smith Papyrus, we are lacking information on the instruments available to surgeons. The famous relief on a box with medical instruments in a Ptolemaic temple in Kom Ombo (fig. 21) comes from an outer enclosure wall,

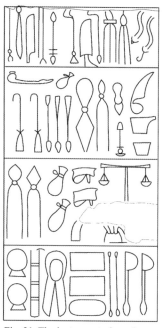

Fig. 21. The instruments from the medical bag of an Egyptian surgeon include a whole range of tongue depressors, hooks, small spoons, blades, knives, pliers, and small vessels. (Roman Period, Temple at Kom Ombo, drawing: H. Vymazalová after Nunn 1996, Fig. 8.2)

which the Roman emperor Trajan (AD 98–117) had built and which was not covered with reliefs until the second half of the second century AD. It accurately depicts the instruments of the Roman imperial period, used not only in Rome itself but also in the provinces, like Egypt (Künzl 1983). The collection of surgical instruments depicted, intended apparently for eye operations (Leca 1971, Pl. XI), is considered by Nunn (1996, 165) also to be later than the dynastic period, so they do not really represent the pharaonic instruments.

A similar depiction is missing from the dynastic period of Egypt, and archaeological excavations have not yet produced a preserved bag with the instruments of an ancient Egyptian physician. However, from other contexts we know of finds of objects of everyday life that could have also been suitably used for minor surgery, yet none of them appears to have been produced exclusively for medical operations.

They include predominantly a knife; surgical interventions are labeled as "knife treatment." In the earliest times, it was a lithic flint knife (Vachala and Svoboda 1989); its sharp edges, acquired by chipping, were used for performing such fine operations as circumcision or depilation until the beginning of Christianity (fig. 22). According to Nunn (1996, 164–65), there were five words for various types of knives, three with a simple determinative for knife, one with the hieroglyphic sign for metal (usually copper). The last knife, in the shape of a swallow's tail *(peseshkef)*, was known from the 'opening of the mouth' ritual (Vachala 2006, 468–70), which Egyptian priests performed above mummies just before burial so the dead would regain the ability to consume food, breathe, speak, and so on (fig. 23). Roth (1992) and Harer (1994) documented the relationship of the *peseshkef* knife to the headrest of the goddess Meskhenet (fig. 24), who attended childbirths, and both came to the opinion that this knife might have been used for cutting the umbilical cord.

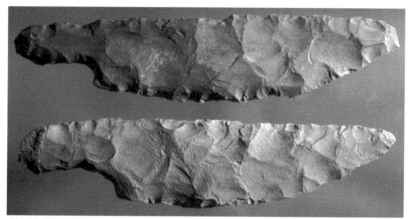

Fig. 22. Flint knives used for cult purposes. (Fifth Dynasty, pyramid complex of Queen Khentkaus II at Abusir, photo: M. Zemina)

Fig. 23. The collection of instruments for the ritual of 'opening the mouth,' which was performed on the mummy just before the funeral to revivify the dead. It included a *peseshkef* knife in the shape of a swallow's tail, cups that were usually made of mountain crystal and obsidian, and other objects. (Fifth Dynasty, pyramid complex of King Neferefre, photo: J. Brodský)

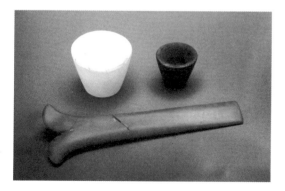

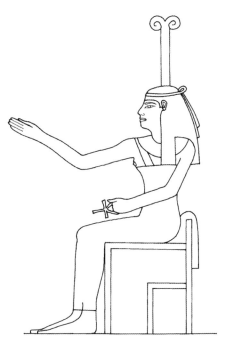

Fig. 24. The goddess Meskhenet, who assisted women in childbirth, was depicted in the form of a woman with the symbol of a cow's uterus on her head. This symbol is reminiscent of the shape of the ritual knife, *peseshkef.* (Eighteenth Dynasty, Hatshepsut's temple at Deir al-Bahari, drawing: J. Malátková after Naville 1896, Pl. LI)

The other commonly used instruments were shepherd's shears, primitive pincers or pliers, lancets, small spoons, tongue depressors, small sticks (probes), and drills and needles of metal (copper, later bronze), wood, or bone (fig. 25).

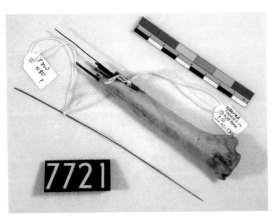

Fig. 25. The instruments of an Egyptian physician evidently included copper needles, which already appear among the archaeological finds from the Predynastic Period. This collection of needles in a bird-bone case comes from the New Kingdom. (Eighteenth Dynasty (?), Petrie Museum of Egyptian Archaeology [UC 7721] at University College London, photo with thanks to the Petrie Museum of Egyptian Archaeology, UCL)

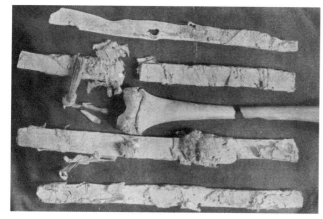

Fig. 26. Wooden splints were to aid the healing of broken bones of the forearm. There are no evident signs of healing on these bones, which indicates that the patient apparently died as a consequence of the injury. (Fifth Dynasty, Naga al-Deir, after Smith 1908, Fig. 3)

Before a surgical operation, physicians usually heated the knife or other instrument to prevent bleeding. They did not realize that in so doing they simultaneously killed pathogenic germs. A hot metal or wooden stick was used for lancing pustules, removing warts, or cauterizing, easing the pain as a secondary effect.

For ritual reasons, the bandages used for wrapping wounds, fractures, and other pathological phenomena had to be made from pure linen, like the bandages used for wrapping mummies. Threads, nets, pads (tampons), or small cushions (rolled linen cylinders) were also made of linen.

For the immobilization of hand-set fractures, splints from the ribs of palm leaves, the bark of some trees, wooden sticks, or reeds were used (Smith 1908) (fig. 26).

Pain relief

In the medical papyri and other literary documents of ancient Egypt, we do not find any description of the course of an ancient Egyptian operation, so we have no idea whether and how Egyptian physicians reduced the pain perception threshold for the pain that accompanied a surgical procedure, or the injury or disease itself. Did the patients have to endure it at the price of great suffering, thanks only to their resistance, which seems admirable to us, from the observation of healed severe pathological processes (Strouhal and Horáčková 2007; Strouhal and Němečková 2009)? Or were there means available to relieve pain (analgesics) or to reduce the perception of pain (narcotics)?

Already in ancient Egypt, the most common stupefying substance, available to broad classes of people, was beer, containing alcohol and produced from fermented bread. The members of the higher social class also often became drunk also with wine, which as the nobler drink accompanied feasts, captured in the reliefs and paintings in the Theban tombs of the New Kingdom (fig. 27). Direct evidence of its use as an intoxicant in Egyptian surgery is so far lacking, but wine and beer appear to have been commonly used as a vehicle to convey a medicine (vehiculum) in a number of recipes, which we shall see in chapter 4, "Mother and Child Care."

Perhaps already from the Old Kingdom (Sullivan 1998, 110), and certainly during the New Kingdom, Egyptians knew the pain-relieving (analgetic), sense-blunting (narcotic), and calming (sedative) effects of the roots, leaves, and fruit of the mandrake (Manniche 1999, 117–19; Reeves 1992, 55–61), which contain atropine and scopolamine. So far, it has not been demonstrated that these plant parts corresponded to some as-yet-unknown medicine in the medical papyri, nor have they been identified in archaeological finds in Egypt. Considering the numerous influences from Mesopotamia, where they were commonly prescribed (Thompson 1923, 59), their use in Egypt can, however, be seriously considered.

Wild-growing poppy was known also in Egypt, apparently already in the Old Kingdom. Whereas in Mesopotamia it was cultivated and used in recipes for pain relief (in the form of suppositories with fat), in Egypt the use of a cultivated form of poppy is not reliably documented until the New Kingdom. Thanks to long-term contacts with Mesopotamia, it seems likely that poppy was imported into Egypt (Sullivan 1998, 111). During the Eighteenth Dynasty, poppy seeds may have also been imported into Egypt, in vessels in the shape of upside-down poppy heads, from Cyprus, where poppies were cultivated on a large scale (Nunn 1996, 156).

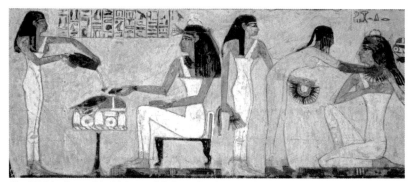

Fig. 27. Members of the higher social class often became drunk on wine at feasts, as shown in the reliefs and paintings in the Theban tombs from the New Kingdom. (Eighteenth Dynasty, tomb of Rekhmire at Sheikh Abd al-Qurna [TT 100], photo: S. Vannini)

Mentions of poppy in medical papyri are rather sporadic. We find its use in Case 41 of the Smith Papyrus; it appears twice also in the Ebers Papyrus (Cases 443 and 782), but not in connection with a surgical procedure. In the analysis of the remnants of the contents of one of the pots from the tomb of the royal architect Kha in Deir al-Medina (TT 8, Eighteenth Dynasty), their narcotic effect was demonstrated by an experiment on frogs, which hence allegedly "identified morphine" (Manniche 1999, 132). Nonetheless, new research has disproved this conclusion (Bisset et al. 1994).

In later periods, poppy was also cultivated in Egypt, and unripe poppy pods were used to acquire an extract with opium, very likely utilized to relieve pain. In the Ptolemaic and Roman Periods, Theban opium became a famous export item (Estes 1989, 152; Schott 1993). Diodorus of Sicily (first century BC) even attributed to Egyptians primacy in the use of opium, "which brings oblivion from all past pain" and "cures fear and sadness" (*Bibliotheca Historica* I 97: 7–8, 333–35).

Whether hemp was used here as a popular remedy for internal, eye, skin, and women's diseases (see chapter 4), as well as for its pain-relieving effect, has not been proved yet (Nunn 1996, 156). The flowers and rhizome of the lotus contain four types of alkaloids, which have a narcotic effect if swallowed or drunk with wine in which the parts of the plants have been macerated. The mere inhalation of the smell of the lotus (fig. 28) was not sufficient for this purpose (Nunn 1996, 157–58).

It seems that it was possible for Egyptian physicians to use some of the above-mentioned means that could reduce the pain threshold of the surgical patient before the procedure. It was naturally still very far from modern narcosis and painless operations.

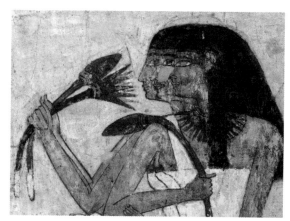

Fig. 28. The inhalation of the scent of lotuses is a frequent subject of depictions in tombs, because for ancient Egyptians, the lotus symbolized resurrection. Women also put lotuses in their hair. (Eighteenth Dynasty, tomb of Rekhmire [TT 100] at Sheikh Abd al-Qurna, photo: S. Vannini)

More difficult was suppressing infections, for which only honey could be used, as it is a bactericide (Estes 1989, 68–70), in combination with hot oil. We have already mentioned the heating of metal instruments before their use for an operation.

Other, often bizarre or disgusting 'medicines,' acting magically or psychotherapeutically (recommended in Case 9 of the Edwin Smith Papyrus, but also in several cases of the surgical treatment in the Ebers Papyrus), were prescribed for calming the patient or alleviating symptoms or pain (palliative care). This was done when the prognosis was hopeless, in order for the patient to receive the help of the gods if it was not within the powers of the physician to help him in his suffering—therefore it would seem that something was being done for the ill person *(ut aliquid fieri videatur)*.

Evidence of surgical operations

We learned about the treatment of wounds with the cases of the Edwin Smith Papyrus. With non-infected wounds, the edges were either drawn together with two linen bands, or the physician proceeded to suture them with a linen-

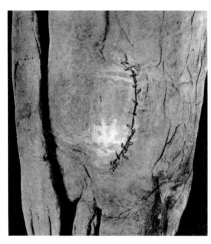

Fig. 29. Evidence of stitches has been preserved, particularly in connection with mummification. After removing the viscera, the hole in the left hypochondrium was closed with rough stitches. Stitches from surgical procedures, however, are attested only in texts. (Twenty-first Dynasty, Egyptian Museum, Cairo, after Smith and Dawson 1924, Fig. 36).

fiber thread. This was done also with the living, not only with mummies, in whose case evidence has been preserved (fig. 29).

If the wound was contaminated—inflamed by a defensive reaction (infection) or purulent—it could not be closed. Its treatment began with the meat of a freshly slaughtered animal, which could be applied to it for only one day. The wound was subsequently washed with hot oil with added honey, to clean it. Only then was it possible to wrap it and bandage it repeatedly.

The paleopathological evidence of serious injuries to the skull, both healing and fresh, was amassed by Pahl (1985–86, 110–29) and compared to the descriptions of the analogous cases 3, 4,

5, 9, 13, 17, and 23 of the Edwin Smith Papyrus. On the other hand, Rösing (1980) studied an extensive collection of skeletons from various periods from the provincial burial grounds in Qubbat al-Hawa on the west bank of the Nile at Aswan. He illustrated the rarity of the paleopathological evidence of medical procedures that would correspond to the descriptions of wounds in the medical papyri.

The find of healed incarcerations of two cervical vertebrae from a Ptolemaic tomb in Saqqara graphically illustrates the description of the same injury in Case 33 of the Edwin Smith Papyrus. Despite the inauspicious prognosis, the elderly man survived this injury, though with severe lifelong disability (Strouhal and Horáčková 2007) (see fig. 14).

Amputations of the hand were associated most likely with military conflicts. However, such cases when the injured in battle survived and returned home were few in Egypt's peaceful times. An exception was violence between individuals, but it is not possible to exclude even curative amputations with life-threatening illnesses or amputations conducted as punishment for thieves. Mainly, however, it is not possible to determine the reason for the amputation with certainty from the remains.

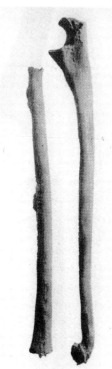

One of the finds shows an amputation above the right wrist of a forty- to fifty-year-old man from the burial ground of the Late to Ptolemaic Period in Abusir. It is revealed by the bend of the lower end of the ulna toward the radius, both ends of which were secondarily broken off. It was here that a bone bridge originally formed during healing by joining the amputated ends of both bones (fig. 30). We can no longer discover the reason for the amputation today (Strouhal and Bareš 1993, 106, Plate 69: 6, fig. 23).

Another amputation, of the big toe of the right foot, on a mummy of an elderly woman from the tomb of Sheikh Abd al-Qurna on the west bank of the Nile at Luxor most likely had a curative reason. The missing phalanx bones of the big toe were replaced after healing by a wooden prosthesis

Fig. 30. One of the Czech archaeological finds shows an amputation above the right wrist of a forty- to fifty-year-old man. (Late–Ptolemaic Period, Abusir, photo: E. Strouhal)

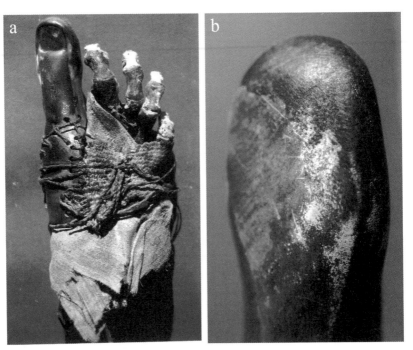

Fig. 31. The amputation of the big toe of the right foot of the mummy of an older woman was probably done for curative purposes. The missing phalanx bones of the big toe were replaced after healing by a wooden prosthesis attached to the first instep bone by a well-thought-out system of strings and bandages to enable movement of the wooden toe (a). Its bottom still has traces of abrasion from walking (b). (Eighteenth Dynasty, tomb of Mery [TT 95] at Sheikh Abd al-Qurna, after Nerlich et al. 2000)

attached at the places of the articulation with the first metatarsus by a well-planned system of strings and bandages, allowing movement of the wooden big toe (fig. 31a). Its bottom still bears traces of abrasion from walking (fig. 31b, Nerlich et al. 2000). It proves not only the surgical operation itself but also the existence of some paramedical employment of bandagers or producers of body prosthetics, who had been associated formerly only with bandaging dead bodies or supplying the missing parts of the bodies during mummification.

Reliefs depicting the victory of the Egyptian armies over enemies contain scenes showing the counting of chopped-off arms or penises of the enemy, piled in heaps. This was not about amputations with live captives but about determining the number of slain opponents. The aim was to overstate their number for propaganda purposes.

Cranial trepanation, a surgery whose execution has not been proved so far in the existing ancient Egyptian written sources, was masterfully described by Mika Waltari in his novel *The Egyptian*. The procedure might have really been performed in that manner, but the novel gives a false idea that it was an entirely common and hence typical surgery in Egypt. This is not the case. A description of trepanation is lacking in the Edwin Smith Papyrus as well as in other written sources. Considering the enormous number of skeletons investigated in Egypt by experts, estimated to be in the thousands, there is an entirely insignificant amount of direct evidence of trepanation as yet.

The conduct of this operation—mainly for the purpose of removing fragments and smoothing the edges of fragmented breaks of the skull bones—was proved only with finds of fourteen complete and nine incomplete (symbolic or entirely healed) trepanations (figs. 32 and 33). In them, a scraping technique was predominantly used, in combination with a cutting method, with the exception of a single case from the Middle Kingdom conducted by drilling. The survival rate for the trepanations was around seventy percent (Pahl 1993, 360–62, fig. 34). Other evidence of similar surgical procedures of ancient Egyptian minor surgery can be expected in the future, as archaeological research advances with the participation of paleopathologists and anthropologists.

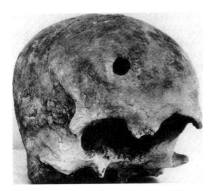 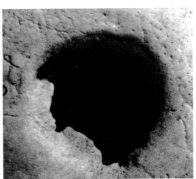

Fig. 32. Scratches on the skull of an adult male are evidence of trepanation. (Twenty-second Dynasty, Medinet Habu, after Pahl 1993, p. 227 Abb. 3/202)

Fig. 33. A healing trepanation on the skull, from the excavations at the cemetery in Tarkhan (First–Second Dynasties, Tarkhan, after Pahl 1993, 221–22)

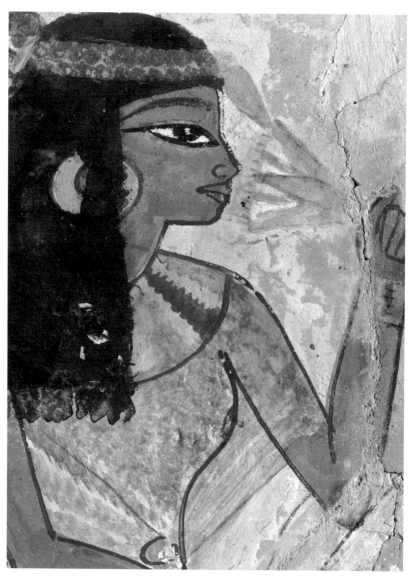

Fig. 34. This appealing depiction of an Egyptian woman is from an Eighteenth Dynasty tomb (Eighteenth Dynasty, tomb of Nakht [TT 52] at Sheikh Abd al-Qurna, photo: S. Vannini)

4

MOTHER AND CHILD CARE

O ther specialized branches of medicine are gynecology, obstetrics, and pediatrics. Today, the first two of these fields are of a surgical nature, and even in pediatrics there is a surgical branch in addition to internal medicine. Although we do not encounter surgical procedures in relation to women and children in the Egyptian sources, we can study this branch of ancient Egyptian medicine in a large group of cases in the preserved texts. Despite the fact that it concerns two different groups of patients suffering from their specific problems, we will deal with them in parallel, because just like in real life, women/mothers are connected with their children, and a large proportion of medical cases recorded in the Egyptian texts concern pregnancy, childbirth, and care of newborns.

In these medical texts, we find methods and means for mother and child care that are intended not only for treating various diseases, but also for treatment during pregnancy and for protection during childbirth and afterward. Many of these cases call on the aid of supernatural powers.

Medical Texts Concerning Women and Children

Cases describing diverse feminine problems and those related to the treatment of children are a component of several medical texts, including the extensive Ebers Papyrus and Edwin Smith "Surgical" Papyrus, which we have discussed in chapter 3. In the majority of these texts, women's cases and children's treatment are mixed with prescriptions for problems of another type, from injuries to various internal ailments.

The synopsis of the papyri and pertinent cases concerning women and children can be found in table 2. The basic information on the individual medical texts, specifying their age, the find circumstances and context, current location, and list of their earlier publications and translations, has been provided in chapter 2.

Table 2. Synopsis of medical texts

Papyrus	Number of Cases	Topic
Kahun	34	women
Ramesseum III, IV	20	women, children
Edwin Smith	1	women
Ebers	62	women, children
Berlin 3038	15	women, children
Carlsberg VIII	7	women
London BM 10059	4	women, children
Berlin 3027	21	women, children
Total Number of Cases	164	

The Kahun Papyrus is the best-known text of the entire group (fig. 35), because it is devoted exclusively to women's issues and includes a whole range of cases of various diseases of women. It is sometimes labeled as a "gynecological papyrus," but the methods of treatment that it describes have little in common with today's concept of gynecology and obstetrics.

The first seventeen cases on the Kahun Papyrus have a unified form comprising the heading "A prescription for a woman suffering . . . ," the determination of the diagnosis "You say of it . . ." (or also "You say of her . . ."), and the prescription "You prepare for her . . ." or "You do with this . . . ." According to the text, not only patently gynecological problems but also manifestations of pain in other parts of the body were put in the context of the female reproductive system. The following eight cases (18–25) are badly damaged and thus difficult to understand. They deal, for example, with distinguishing between fertile and infertile women, inducing conception, or contraceptive means. Another group of cases (26–32) concern determining pregnancy, often

Fig. 35. The Kahun Gynecological Papyrus has been only partially preserved. The numerous gaps in the text make some of the cases difficult to understand. (Twelfth Dynasty, Petrie Museum of Egyptian Archaeology [UC 32057], photo: with thanks to the Petrie Museum of Egyptian Archaeology, UCL)

in connection with swollen breasts. The final group (33–34) includes a case of toothache during pregnancy and a case of painful urination.

Papyrus Carlsberg VIII captures only cases related to women, but it has been preserved in a very poor condition and therefore is not so well known. It seems, however, that in this text the cases had a rather unified form, with a title presenting the purpose of the examination and a description of the acts that were to be carried out for the woman. The six partially preserved cases provide the instructions for judging the fertility of a woman and determining the state of pregnancy as well as the gender of the unborn child.

Determining the fertility of a woman is also the topic in the group of cases on the verso of Papyrus Berlin 3038 (193–198) that are introduced with the title "How to recognize a woman who will give birth . . . ." Case 192 describes a contraceptive method and Case 199 a pregnancy test, which is often interpreted as determining the sex of the child in the mother's womb. On the recto of the same papyrus, we find among the many other cases a group assigned for the treatment of children (13–18, 30). The cases are very brief and are presented by the title "A remedy to . . ." or merely "Another (remedy)." This is followed by a brief description of the preparation and method of application of the medicine.

The fragments of papyrus found in the Ramesseum contain cases related to both groups of patients, women and children. We find them mixed together in Ramesseum III, in two sections, A and B, and in Ramesseum IV. They are instructions for easing childbirth, contraceptive methods, approaches for sick children, and also for assuring protection of the child. Rather than medicine, most cases use magic, whose effect from today's point of view is more psychotherapeutic.

Only one case in the "surgical" Edwin Smith Papyrus, which was analyzed in detail in chapter 3, relates specifically to women and describes the treatment of menstrual problems. It is Case 20 on the verso, at the very end of the text, which was added after the surgical cases by another scribe.

The Ebers Papyrus is the most voluminous of all of the preserved medical papyri. On 110 pages of text, a total of 877 cases from various areas of medicine are recorded. Chapter 3 describes the cases of surgical treatment of some diseases. The cases related to women's problems (783–839) include instructions for easing childbirth and care for the mother after childbirth,

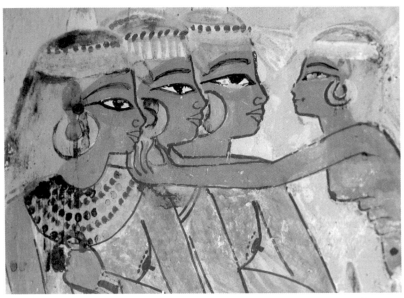

Fig. 36. Girls and women were a popular motif of the depictions in many Theban tombs. In this scene, a very young girl is serving three women who are attending a banquet. (Eighteenth Dynasty, tomb of Nakht [TT 52] at Sheikh Abd al-Qurna, photo: M. Megahed)

prescriptions for breast treatment, and also for the treatment of various gyne-cological problems. In addition, the treatment methods in Cases 169 and 174 are related to women. Children's diseases are dealt with by Cases 262, 272–283, which provide the instructions for urinary problems, and 782, offering a solution for a child that is crying bitterly.

The medical texts concerning female and child patients include both instructions and prescriptions intended to treat the problems whose cause was known and curable, and methods based on magic, which were to help where the knowledge of Egyptian doctors and healers on the causes of the diseases failed. This general principle is very typical for Egyptian medicine by and large and reveals much to us about domestic religious practices, as well as the superstition that reigned in Egyptian society.

Magical methods for the protection of a woman during pregnancy have been preserved on the papyrus from the British Museum (BM 10059), but particular attention should be paid to the text on Papyrus Berlin 3027, which is known as the *Book for Mother and Child*. It contains several medical pre-scriptions, but its principal part consists of magical incantations that were to help protect the woman during pregnancy, childbirth, and puerperium, and also the child after its birth and in infancy, when it was threatened by a wide range of illnesses and infections, whose causes were often not understood by Egyptian physicians. This papyrus is usually not included in the collection of classic medical texts, because the treatment methods described in it are based on magical incantations against unfriendly forces, which supposedly evoked various diseases according to religious concepts, not on rational knowledge and means of scientific medicine of the time. The incantations recorded in the *Book for Mother and Child*, however, evidence the activity of magicians (for example, *sau*) (Grapow 1956, 94) in expelling diseases or their instigators (exorcism) and the usage of protective means (amulets) to prevent future danger. It is necessary to imagine the possibilities of that time, when it was not in the powers of rational medicine to cure all of the maladies suffered by the ill or injured, in this case mothers and children. The aid of supernatural powers based on the elements of the universal religious world-view of the ancient Egyptians was therefore welcome. These methods can be compared to the exorcism of evil spirits by the Christian Church or to the deep psychoanalysis of modern psychology and psychiatry.

The words uttered by the magician had a positive psychotherapeutic effect on the sick, who either had not had successful treatments with real physicians or did not have access to them. The incantations from the *Book for Mother and Child* also contain some terms reflecting the anatomical knowledge of that time. On the other hand, the translations of the names of some of the symptoms mentioned still evade our knowledge. The cases of twenty-one incantations from the *Book for Mother and Child* can be divided into four categories: exorcism for children in danger and the production of protective amulets, prescriptions for sick children, protection in childbirth, and incantations for ensuring the quality of breast milk.

The Ingredients of Remedies for Women and Children

Unlike in the treatment of the surgical cases, which relied predominantly on several main ingredients (honey, oil, raw meat), in the treatment of women and children we encounter a great number of various medicinal preparations. The texts mention a wide range of ingredients, which can be of mineral, plant, or animal origin. The ingredients are usually named one by one, along with the instructions for their preparation. They can be simply mixed, ground, mashed, crushed, pulverized, firmed, cooked, cooled, strained, and so on. Some of these ingredients remain unknown to us so far, and so it is not possible to judge their medical effect. In such cases, we place in the text a phonetic transcription of the Egyptian name of the substance.

Units

In the production of healing mixtures, their amount is in many cases specified, using ancient Egyptian units of volume. The most common unit is *hin*, which was also the name of a vessel that had a standard volume and was used as a measuring cup. In the texts, the amount of a certain ingredient is sometimes specified as "*x hin*"; other times it is stated that the ingredient is to be "served in *hin*." The meaning is the same in both cases, because the basic information here is the amount that should be used for the production of the medicine, measured with a uniform measuring vessel.

In some cases, the amount of the ingredients is marked by the numeral 1, as in "trigonella 1, honey 1." The number here can represent the amount of 1 *hin* or simply "an equal amount" of both mentioned ingredients.

Another very popular unit of volume for the ancient Egyptians was the grain measure *(heqat)*, which corresponded to 4.8 liters and for whose parts they used special marks different from the common Egyptian numerals (Vymazalová 2006, 19). It was used particularly for measuring grains, and sometimes also liquids. Table 3 contains a brief synopsis of the basic units and their equivalents.

Table 3. Ancient Egyptian measurements

1 grain measure *(heqat)* = 4.8 l
1 *hin* = 1/10 grain measure = 0.48 l = 480 ml
1/2 grain measure = 2.4 l
1/4 grain measure = 1.2 l
1/8 grain measure = 600 ml
1/16 grain measure = 300 ml
1/32 grain measure = 150 ml
1/64 grain measure = 5 *ro* = 75 ml
1 *ro* = 1/320 grain measure = 15 ml

Ingredients from the kitchen

The foodstuff ingredients particularly included beer *(henqet)*, sometimes specified as sweet beer or high-quality beer. The most common Egyptian beer was produced from barley, through fermentation from flat yeast cakes finely ground in water (Helck 1971), and it was more nutritious than alcoholic. Sometimes, the sediments or dregs *(tahet)* of beer or even its foam were used in medical preparations. The beer *djesret* was stronger than common beer. Beer was added to various prescriptions; in some cases, it could lower the pain threshold (for example, in childbirth). Likewise wine *(irep)* was used for the same purpose. In medical mixtures, we also find barley and wheat, which were the basic grains of the Egyptian diet, as well as flour or yeast.

In many cases, honey *(bit)*, which has antibacterial and fungicidal effects, was used for treatment and could thus help prevent infections. It was further used in preparations against conception, where it acted as a spermicide.

Some of the ingredients that we encounter in the preserved texts are entirely unknown, and not even the cases themselves reveal anything on their character. For instance, the expressions *mesta* and *khawy* mark some kind of liquids, about whose preparation, however, we know nothing. The meaning of the expression *weshet* is also unknown.

Ingredients of mineral origin

The ingredients of mineral origin included water, dew, clay or mud from the Nile, and a great number of minerals. In the prescriptions, salt *(hemat)* often appeared, which could add flavor to the medicinal mixtures but also had an osmotic effect, and a warm solution of salt was slightly emetic. Some cases required salt from the Delta (Lower Egypt), which was likely sea salt acquired by evaporation. Natron *(hesmen)*, or also a paste from natron, was used less often. The popular ingredients further included ochre *(sety)* or red ochre *(menshet)*, galenite *(mesdemet)*, and malachite *(wadju)*, the latter two likewise used as black and green eye makeup, respectively.

Some of the mineral ingredients remain unknown, for instance *kesenty*, *hetem*, or *nehdet*. The ingredient called "great protection" *(sa-wer)* was most likely of mineral nature (Hannig 1997, 655), although according to some specialists it could be a type of resin (Barns 1956, 16).

Ingredients of herbal origin

The ingredients of herbal origin included various types of herbs as well as woody plants, fruits, berries, and grains. The herbs included, for instance, sedge *(iaru)* and rush *(sut)*, both the male and female plants of each, reed *(nebit)*, nut grass *(giu)*, whose rhyzomes or tubers *(wah)* are also called earth almonds, sorghum *(mimi)*, flax *(mehy)*, and pellitory, or Spanish chamomile *(shames)*. In medical science, the papyrus plant *(mehyet)*, which grew in the Nile Delta, was also used. Its stalks grew as high as five meters and were used in many areas of production. Potamogeton *(nesha)* had an astringent and refreshing effect. Trigonella *(hemat)* contains a great quantity of vitamins, and its seeds allegedly support lactation and facilitate the healing of inflammations. Yellow sweet clover *(afay)* restrains the activity of the smooth muscle tissue and thus has a favorable effect on digestion. It also works against flatulence and limits blood coagulation.

Flavor was given to medicinal mixtures by coriander *(shau)*, Roman cumin *(tepnen)*, or fennel *(besbes)*, all of which, moreover, had a positive effect on digestion. The identity of the term *djaret* is questionable. Some experts identify it as colocynth, while others consider it the pulp of the pods of the carob tree, which is also known as St. John's Bread and works as a lubricant and for soothing (a demulcent). Henbane *(pesedj)* could have had a more serious effect, but since it is a dangerous narcotic, it is likely that only one of its parts was used (Barns 1956, 26). From the lotus *(seshen)*, a part called *khau*, which is not more clearly defined, appears in the texts. The flowers of the lotus contain narcotic alkaloids soluble in alcohol. The term *shemshemet* is usually interpreted as hemp, widely used in many areas of craft production; however, it has not been proved that Egyptian healers were aware of the effects of the substances that cannabis contains. Some experts consider *shemshemet* to be sesame (Germer 2008, 133). In the preparations, there further appears poppy *(shepen)*, whose seeds contain a very small amount of morphine, a narcotic analgesic. The castor oil plant *(kaka)* works as a laxative and also aids healing, but in greater amounts can induce death. The same effects, as well as the danger, are provided by bryony *(khasyt)*.

In the case of woody plants, the recipes listed a certain specific part, for example leaves, fruit, or sawdust, but at other times only the general name of the tree was given, and hence the producer of the medicine had to know which part of the plant to use. The popular ingredients included catclaw acacia *(shendjet)*, which has astringent effects, or parts of the palm tree *(beneret)*, sycamore *(nehet)*, and also the myrtle *(khet-des)*, whose leaves, flowers, and fruit act astringently and antiseptically. From the earliest periods, cedar *(ash)* was imported from Lebanon, and in medical science cedar resin *(adj-ash)* and particularly cedar oil *(sefet)* were used, the latter of which has antiseptic effects and works as a diuretic and against flatulence (a carminative) as well. The same and moreover tonic (stimulating) effect is provided by juniper berry *(wan)*, which was brought from the Sinai or Asia Minor. Incense *(senetjer)* and myrrh *(antyu)*, the resins of rare trees, had great importance, and not only in medicine. Resin *(hedju)* was used in the preparation of various ointments. The prescriptions also list a tree or fruits of the *ished*, whose precise meaning we do not know, but it might be the *Balanites aegyptiaca* (desert date) or Persea. From the seeds of the moringa or benzolive tree *(bak)*, an oil was obtained that had an anti-inflammatory effect. Medical science likewise used the leaves of the cinnamon tree *(hekenu)* and related types of trees, which are labeled with the historical designation malabathrum.

The preparations administered to the Egyptian patient further contained various fruits and tubers. They could be fruits like the date *(bener)* in dried, mashed, or fresh form or in the form of a date purée *(semeret)*; watermelon *(bededu-ka)*; or muskmelon *(shespet, shebet)*.

The cleansing of the system could be aided by onions *(hedju)*, whose juice is a natural antibiotic, diuretic, and expectorant, and by garlic *(kheten)*, which has antibacterial effects. Celery *(matet)* and wild carrot *(kheper-wer)*, whose high content of vitamins was undoubtedly beneficial to one's health, were added to medicines as well. Pine nuts *(pery-sheny)*, peas *(tehu)*, or beans *(iuryt)* appear sporadically in the prescriptions. The seed of the vitex *(saamu)* supposedly helps to relieve menstrual cramps.

The texts mention a wide range of plant names whose meaning we do not yet know. An interesting name has been given to the plant "hyena ear" *(mesdjer hedj-ret)*. The plant *iba* is sometimes identified as the jujuba, but this determination is hardly verifiable. The same applied to the plant *inek* or perhaps *innek*, which was sometimes considered to be horseweed or thyme (Nunn 1996, 154). In the medical prescriptions, we also encounter the unknown plants *ibu, ihu, wam, pakh-seryt, niaia, nebu, heny-ta, khesau, sar, shena, ketket,* and *debyt*. The fruits of the *iwehu*, the fruits of the *shasha*, the seeds of the grass *seneb*, or a powder of the plant *tjun* were used as well. Some part of the plant was labeled as *khenesh*. A decoction of medicinal herbs was called *hesa* and used as an infusion *(hesa shebeb)* or fermented *(hesa awayt)*, but the texts do not mention its precise composition.

Ingredients of animal origin

An ingredient in many of the preparations was oil *(merhet)*, sometimes more precisely identified as fresh oil *(merhet maat)* and white oil *(merhet hedjet)*. Particularly in the treatment of children, milk *(irtet)*, mainly cow's but sometimes also donkey's milk, was used. Human milk from the breast of a mother of a male child was highly appreciated as a magical means and for treatment. The instructions also mention milk fat *(mehwy* or *mehut)* or "milk fat" from fresh oil, which might refer to a sediment taken from oil *(mehwy n merhet mat)*.

The magical sphere *(Dreckapotheke)* included a whole range of disgusting substances, like blood *(senef)*, mainly animal blood. One case required human blood, namely the first menstrual blood. Likewise animal urine could be added to the medicinal mixtures. In many preparations, dung *(hes)* of various animals was used, particularly of crocodile and hippopotamus, but also fly droppings. In two cases, even human feces were required.

Various animal parts or organs were added into medicines and particularly magical remedies, for instance bull bile, spinal cord or marrow, ass and turtle livers or other parts of a turtle's body, dried swallow liver, pig liver or even pig or bull brain, bone marrow, the spine of the Nile bass, parts of the sacred fish *abedju*, and beetles. Magical power was allegedly found in the feathers of black swallows, the hair of a fair donkey, beetles, or a cooked mouse as well. Great importance in medical science and magic was ascribed also to the placenta, which was sometimes considered as a double of the newborn individual and after birth was dried and kept as a talisman.

Sundry other ingredients

A great number of recommended medical methods included magical acts like the production of amulets, magically effective tampons, and so on. In such cases, bundles of plant fibers, pieces of cloth, or linen yarn were often used for the production. Statuettes made of clay or wax, faience balls, or beads of various colors had a magical effect. In one case, even an inscribed (used) papyrus scroll was used, at other times tar oakum or potsherds.

Translation of the Texts

Editorial note: Round brackets ( ) mark contemporary additions for better comprehension of the text. Square brackets [ ] mark restorations of the text that originally were in it but have not been preserved. The words that appear in red ink on the papyri are set in bold in this edition. The translation also reflects the variability of ancient Egyptian terminology. For the labeling of the individual parts of female genitalia, we have used a variety of synonymous expressions, which correspond to the various terms in ancient Egyptian. Most of the cases in the medical papyri are numbered in an ordinal system. The exceptions to this are the cases from the Ramesseum Papyri, which are distinguished by the lines in the text. This labeling is the standard used in specialized literature; therefore, we observe it also in this publication.

Kahun Papyrus

Case Kahun 1: 1–5

Examination of [a woman] aching [in both of her eyes] that she cannot see and has pain in her neck.

You should say of [it: it is discharges] of the uterus in both of her eyes.

You should treat this: fumigate her with incense and fresh oil, fumigate with it her womb, fumigate her eyes with the shank of an oriole, make her eat fresh ass liver.

Case Kahun 2: 5–8

Examination of a woman aching in her uterus when moving.

You should say of it: What is that you smell?

When she tells you: I smell roast, **you should say of it:** it is effusion of the uterus. **You should treat this:** fumigate her with everything that she smells like a roast.

Case Kahun 3: 8–12

Examination of a woman who has pain in her rectum, her pubic region, and both of her inner thighs.

You should say of it: it is discharges of the uterus.

You should treat this: earth almonds 1/64 (grain measure), fruits of the *shasha* 1/64 (grain measure), cow milk 1 *hin*; boil, cool, and mix together. Drink for four mornings.

Case Kahun 4: 12–15

Examination of a woman (suffering) in her pubic region, her womb, and around her womb between her buttocks.

You should say of it: large swelling after birth.

You should treat this: fresh oil 1 *hin*, pour over [her] womb and her [. . .].

Case Kahun 5: 15–20
Examination of a woman aching in her teeth and with pain in her gums (that) she cannot [open] her mouth.

You should say of it: it is toothache (caused by) the uterus.

You should treat this: fumigate her with oil and incense in one vessel, (then) pour over her [. . .] the urine of a fair ass the day after it passed it. When she has pain in her pubic region from her navel to her buttocks, it is incurable.

Case Kahun 6: 20–22
Examination [of a woman] aching in all of her limbs and in both eye sockets.

You should say of it: it is a constriction of the uterus; she must not drink beer at all [. . .] soon after birth.

You should treat this: purée with water 1 (portion). Drink for [. . .] mornings.

Case Kahun 7: 23–25
Examination of a woman having pain in both of her legs and feet after walking.

You should say of it: it is discharges of the uterus.

You should treat this: smear both of her feet and legs with mud until she recovers.

Case Kahun 8: 25–27
Examination of a woman having pain in her neck, her pubic region, and both of her ears so much that she cannot hear a word.

You should say of it: it is cramps of the uterus.

You should treat this: the same prescription as for removing the detritus of the uterus.

Case Kahun 9: 27–29
Examination of a woman having pain in her womb and all of her limbs as if beaten.

You should say of it: it is [. . .] of the womb.

You should treat this: (she should) eat oil until she recovers.

Case Kahun 10: 30–34
Examination of a woman having pain when urinating as if [. . .] urine polluted.

You should say of it: it is discharges of the uterus.

You should treat this: beans, pine nuts, and the *mut* part of nutgrass, grind fine, with a *hin* of diluted beer and boil. Drink for four mornings. She should spend a day and a night fasting; in the morning, drink 1 *hin* of the same and spend the day fasting until breakfast time comes.

Case Kahun 11: 34–36

Examination of a bed-bound woman who (cannot) stretch and shakes it (the bed).
You should say of it: it is clenching of the uterus.
You should treat this: make her drink 2 *hin* of *khawy* and vomit it at once.

Case Kahun 12: 36–40

Examination of a woman having pain in both of her legs.
You should apply to it fine linen strips soaked in myrrh [. . .] pleasant no matter what she does, she has recovered. When [. . .] comes, it is [. . .] of the uterus.
You should treat] this: milk fat of fresh oil; pour over her [. . .] place myrrh on her [. . .] after this has been done.

Case Kahun 13: 40–47

Examination [of a woman having pain in] both of her legs and one side of her [. . .].
You should say of it: [it is] a bending [of the uterus].
You should treat this: pine nuts, vitex, part *mut* of nutgrass, [. . .] side on which it hurts and make her lie on it. When [. . .] returns, [. . .] she chews two and [. . .] two [. . .] divided in her [. . .] When she passes [. . .] when she has done everything [. . .] swollen. You should place your finger on it; if you find it firm [. . .] in the uterus, it is incurable.

Case Kahun 14: 47–49

Examination of a woman who is thirsty [. . .]
You should do with this: fermented decoction 1/64 (grain measure), [. . .] a fermented herbs decoction [. . .] entirely.

Case Kahun 15: 49–50

Examination of a woman whose pubic region is swollen [. . .].
You should do with this: malachite 1/64 (grain measure); finely grind and boil with a unit of cow's milk, milk [fat . . .] three [days].

Case Kahun 16: 51–54

Examination of a woman having pain in all of her limbs and both of [her] eye sockets [. . .] the disease *kemet*.
You should say of it: it is the disease *kemet* of the uterus.
You should treat this: oil [. . .], *ished* fruits, grapes, sycamore fruit, *iwehu* fruits, pine nuts [. . .]; finely grind and boil. Drink it for three days.

Case Kahun 17: 54–59

Examination of a woman bleeding [. . .] placenta and has pain in her head, her mouth, and palm of her hand.

You should say of it: [. . .]

You should treat this: smear the ground for her and place on it dregs of sweet beer [. . .]. If everything does not come out of her, you should place pressed dates on top on the dregs [. . .], make her sit on it. If everything does not come out of her, you should make [. . .] boil [. . .] cooled and make her drink it [. . .]. If, however, blood or pus comes out, it is [. . .]

Case Kahun 18: 1–2

Another (prescription) for revealing [. . .] **from** [. . .] a half scoop of milk, [. . .] scoop [. . .]; solidify and pour over her womb.

Case Kahun 19: 2–3

Determining the baby in the uterus of a woman. When a month returns to a month and [. . .] enters [. . .] failure [. . .]

Case Kahun 20: 3–6

[When a woman] is affected by a prescription for conception, after discontinuing the return [. . .] grind finely, strain through a cloth into a fermented herb decoction, pour milk fat [. . .], incense, fresh oil [. . .], dates, and sweet beer; place inside a pot on a fire. You should fumigate [. . .] with a mouth cleaner.

Case Kahun 21: 6

Preventing [conception]: crocodile dung, crush with fermented herb decoction, dip [. . .]

Case Kahun 22: 7

Another prescription: a *hin* of honey, pour over her womb. To be done (also) with a natron solution.

Case Kahun 23: 7–8

Another [. . .] with fermented herb decoction; pour over her womb.

Case Kahun 24: 8–9

This is for removing toothaches (caused) by uterus: a date-palm stem and [. . .], mash thoroughly in sweet beer [. . .], make her sit on it with her legs apart.

Case Kahun 25: 9–11

Examination of a woman with fever [. . .] both her eyes are bleary. Wild carrot grated in a part of *mesta* drink, pour [. . .] for four mornings. You should make her sit in water of [. . .] and water of a lake, place [. . .]

Case Kahun 26: 12–14

Determining a woman who will conceive from one who will not: you should [. . .] fresh oil with [. . .], you should [. . .] it. If the vessels on her breast are distended, you should say of her: this is one who will give birth. If you find them limp, you should say of her: she will give birth later. If you however find them like the skin [. . .]

Case Kahun 27: 15–17

Another instance: you should make her sit on the ground smeared with dregs of sweet beer, put fruit, dates [. . .] [If] she vomits, she will give birth, (and) also every ejection that comes from her mouth, each (means) a birth [. . .] But if she does not vomit, she will never give birth.

Case Kahun 28: 17–19

Another instance: you should place onion tubers in [her] body [. . .] it there [. . .] [If] you find it in it, you should say of her: she will give birth. If you do not find [. . .] her nose [. . .] she will [never give birth].

Case Kahun 29: 19–20

Another instance: you should pull her by her lip, your fingertips on her shoulder. [If] it hurts [. . .] [If] it does not hurt, she will never give birth.

Case Kahun 30: 20–23

Another instance: This calf of Horus [. . .] I am on [. . .] Horus, and vice versa. Go down to the place where you [. . .]
   [This incantation] is said [. . .]
   If (it) comes out of her nostrils, she will give birth.
   If (it) comes out of her womb, she will give birth.
   If then [. . .] [. . . she will] never [give birth].

Case Kahun 31: 23–24

Another instance: if you see that her face is fresh, with freshness but you find something on her like [. . .]
   [. . .] But if you saw anything on her eyes, she will never give birth.

Case Kahun 32: 24–25

Determining the one who will conceive [. . .]
[. . .] like that finger on the shoulder.

Case Kahun 33: 25–26

Preventing toothache of a woman [. . .] beans, grind with [. . .] on her gums on the day she gives birth. [It is] really effective for driving out toothaches, a million [times].

Case Kahun 34: 27–28

[. . .] **a woman with pain when urinating.** If the urine comes out [. . .] she will recognize it, she will be like that forever.

Papyri from the Ramesseum

Case Ramesseum III.A ll. 1–2

[. . .] **child:** great protection, give him [. . .] in a *hin*. Make him drink it all. If [. . .] excrete because of constipation [. . .]

Case Ramesseum III.A ll. 7–8

When you examine a woman with pain in her legs and her feet, you should say of [it . . .]
You should prepare for her a remedy [. . .] carob and muskmelon; grind finely and mix with [. . .]

Case Ramesseum III.A l. 8

Making a woman urinate [. . .]

Case Ramesseum III.A ll. 9

Driving away thirst in a child [. . .]

Case Ramesseum III.A ll. 30–31

Correcting urination [. . .]
[. . .] reed, mix with settled beer and *khawy* drink; grind finely and drink up by a man; (to a child,) give [. . .]

Case Ramesseum III.B ll. 10–11

Making a child who does not suck accept (the breast):
Swallow! says Horus. Chew! says Seth. Indeed [. . .] was given to you [. . .]

Case Ramesseum III.B ll. 12–14

[. . .] in a child or in a man:

salt, *weshet*, [. . .] Oh you who seek ropes before you, do not make worried this heart of mine, *ib*, and this heart of mine, *haty* [. . .]

[. . .] roll (it) to the left, dip it in a decoction, tie a knot on it, and give to a child or to an adult man.

Case Ramesseum III.B ll. 14–17

Quenching the thirst of a child:

Your hunger has been removed [. . .] your thirst [has been removed] by (the god) Agebuer to the sky (like) the *pakh*-bird. It is your thirst in my fist, it is your hunger in my fist [. . .] (the goddess) Hesat [. . .] her breast is in your mouth. Your mouth is (like) the mouth of the *khabesu*-bird on the outflow of Osiris. You do not eat your hunger, you do not drink [your thirst], your throat has not been struck dumb.

A man recites this incantation above a piece of soil, placed in cloth [. . .] make in [. . .]

Case Ramesseum III.B ll. 19–20

Quenching the thirst of a man or child:

[. . . leave] overnight in water; take out in the morning, pound, strain through [cloth], and give (it) to him in a *hin*.

Case Ramesseum III.B ll. 20–23

Driving away *baa*. What is said as a spell:

Come [. . .] Nut [. . .] I do not know it, do not say my name. Attend (?) that it is pleasing in all for this lord Horus, her son, when the disease *baa* is told: Beware! This is urge that measures the filling of the mouth. The one that has come to drive away, to drive away hunger [. . .]

[. . .] acacia, roll (it up) to the left and give to the child on its neck. It is the driving away of the *baa*-disease.

Case Ramesseum III.B ll. 23–34

[. . .] It is I who come from the marshes [. . .] Isis, Divine: I hit my temples, I tousled my hair when I found my son Horus, his heart weary, his lips pale, and both of his knees weak after he drank up *baa*, which was in my bosom, [the bitterness of my breast.] Sit down to [. . .] Isis, says Horus. Flow out wicked *baa* in this name of yours *baa*, you that suck the heart and cause weakness in both knees of whomever you reside in. Come to the people with me, my mother, says Horus: (also you) sister of my mother, Nephthys, to the place where the wet nurses and servants of Nut are, who will tell us what they have done for their children. Thus, we will do according to (this) example for our children [. . .] Isis, Divine, with Nephthys: I have come because of my son Horus, whose heart is weary and whose both knees are weak [. . . after he drank up] *baa*, which was in my bosom, an evil substance that was in my breast.

His amulets shall be put on seven straws of flax spun and woven by a woman who has (just) given birth; bring a nestling of a swallow; the eyes shall be painted [. . .] with galenite [. . .] this child with his mother. His *baa* (belongs to) the swallow.

Recite this incantation over the seven straws of flax, spun and woven by a woman who has given birth. Tie seven knots in it and give to the child on his neck. You should bring the swallow [. . .] in its throat [. . .].

Case Ramesseum IV.A ll. 2–4

[. . .] **having pain in the pubic region** and having pain in sex and things do not cease [. . .] [When you palpate her] loins and you find her [. . .]

Case Ramesseum IV.C ll. 1–2

[. . .] **on cakes** [. . .] **every day and make the woman swallow.**

Case Ramesseum IV.C ll. 2–3

Preventing conception in a woman.

You (should) **say:** crocodile dung [. . .] soak a wad, apply to the mouth of her womb [. . .]

Case Ramesseum IV.C ll. 6–7

Driving away [*neshu*] of a child:

henbane [. . .], Lower Egyptian barley [. . .] [. . .] Boil with a decoction; to be drunk by the child.

Case Ramesseum IV.C ll. 12–15

Making a child evacuate [. . .]

[Come to me] gods, says Isis, the Divine, and make sure the fire left. The child [. . .] of the mother [. . .] the mother as a guide. Flow out, you painful excrement, leave onto the ground!

Recite [. . .] with fresh ink on the belly of the child.

Case Ramesseum IV.C II. 15–16

Making a protection for a child on the day of his birth [. . .]
a piece of dung from him after he has come out of the womb of his mother
[. . .]

Case Ramesseum IV.C II. 17–24

Another thing that can be done for him on the day of his birth:
a piece of its placenta with [. . .] pulp with milk and give (it) to him during the day. If he vomits it, he will die. If he [swallows] it, he will live.

Then you should say: Your grace . . . brought for it (?) without incantations [. . .] next to this tree *ished* of Osiris. Oh you that have created and have made the womb, [. . .] of the dead which has intercourse, impregnates, and embraces during the night and kisses during the day. Do not have intercourse [. . . with] this woman, do not fraternize with her, do not do (to her) any bad or evil thing, your nose [. . .] [. . .] your [. . .] are bleary, do not do any bad or evil thing.

Recite the words above a figurine [of a child], fumigate the woman on it. When it is pleasant, the childbirth will be good. When it is unpleasant, the childbirth [will be bad].

Case Ramesseum IV.C II. 25–28

[. . .] Hemen his mother Isis; he made [his] sister [Nephthys] pregnant with a daughter [. . .] Shu, Shu! Tefnut, Tefnut! Geb, Geb! Osiris, this is the lath of the builders of the temple of (the god) Ha in [. . .] You have brought into being for me this boy [. . .] born of this woman [. . .] **which has happened before.**

Case Ramesseum IV.C II. 28–30

(How) to drive out (a child) from its mother.
My mother is like [. . .] like Nephthys. What is it that he sees on the top of the head of the Great (goddess ?) [. . .] Come out on the ground [. . .]

Recite this incantation over a bit of ointment, spread on the top of the head of a woman who is giving birth.

Edwin Smith Papyrus
Case Smith verso 20: 20,13–21,3

If you examine a woman having pain in her stomach, whose menstruation has not started, and you find something on the upper side of her navel. You should say of it: it is stagnation of her blood in her womb.
You should prepare for her: the plant *wam* 1/16 (grain measure), oil 1/8, sweet beer 1/8 (grain measure); cook and drink for four days.

Also prepare for her (a remedy) for having blood leave: cedar oil, cumin, galenite, and aromatic myrrh; grind together, spread on her womb many times. You should add the plant "hyena's ear" to the oil.

When she later begins to bleed, you should rub and spread it on her pelvic region many times. You should place the myrrh and incense between her thighs so the smoke enters her vagina.

Ebers Papyrus

Case Ebers 169: 34,14–34,15
Another (prescription for removing magic substances from a person): powder from dates, add to oil and put it in the vessel *shebet*, put it on the fire and add yeast. (Give it) to eat to a woman whose belly refuses.

Case Ebers 174: 35,2–35,4
Another: the plant *ibu* **1/64**, coriander **1/16**, sorghum **1/16**, fruits *shasha* **1/8**, pellitory **1/16**. Cook with honey **half 1/64** (grain measure); (give it) to eat to a woman when she goes to sleep.

Case Ebers 262: 48,22–49,2
Another (remedy) for making a child pass the accumulation of urine that is in his belly: a used papyrus scroll, cooked in oil; smear (it) on his belly to correct his urination.

Case Ebers 272 bis: 49,18–49,21
Another (remedy) for correcting urination of a child: pith from a reed, completely grind with sweet beer, the dregs of the drink *khawy*. To drink by the woman in a *hin* so that it is given to the child.

Case Ebers 273: 49,21–50,2
What is done for a child suffering from bedwetting: faience, cook until soft (and form) into balls. If the child is big, he swallows it as a medicine. If he is in diapers, pulp it for him in the milk from his wet nurse to drink for four days.

Case Ebers 782: 93,3–93,5
Remedy for driving away the excessive cries of a child: poppy seeds, fly droppings that were on the wall. Mix together, strain, (and give to the child) to eat for four days. It will stop.

Concerning an excessive scream: it is a child who constantly screams.

Case Ebers 783: 93,6–93,8
The beginning of the remedy that is prepared for women and given to prevent a woman from conceiving for one, two, or three years:

kaa of acacia, carob, and dates, grind finely with a *hin* of honey, wet a fiber wad in it, and place it in her vagina.

Case Ebers 784: 93,9–93,10
A remedy for preventing hurting when a woman is urinating:

salt from the Delta 1/16, milk fat 1/8, sweet beer 1/16 1/64 (grain measure), honey 1/64 (grain measure); pour into the rectum.

Case Ebers 785: 93,10–93,11
Another (remedy) for cooling the rectum:

moringa oil 1, oil 1, carob juice 1, honey 1; pour into the rectum.

Case Ebers 786 + 787: 93,11–93,17
Another doing for one (woman) passing clots:

pieces of mud from the Nile that have not been exposed to light, place (them) on white ground, splatter with a lot of water, (and leave) overnight. You should have a new bowl and a new pot, both filled with water, exposed to the dew overnight. You should splatter those pieces again at the rising of the morning gods (= stars) and make the woman sit on it for many days. You should have a new pot brought filled with oil, make the woman sit on it for four days.

Case Ebers 788: 93,17–93,18
Determination of spoiled milk:

you should see that its smell is like the smell of fish.

Case Ebers 789: 93,18–93,20
A remedy for causing the placenta of a woman to leave into its place:

sawdust of cedar, put into the dregs (of beer), spread a cloth cushion. You should make her sit on it.

Case Ebers 790: 93,20–93,21
Another: clay, which has been sprayed (?), toughen with honey; spread it to the pubic region of the woman.

Case Ebers 791: 93,21-94,1
Another: a tar oakum that is in a boat, pulp into the dregs of excellent beer and give it to her to drink up.

Case Ebers 792: 94,2-94,3
Another: ochre 1, strengthen with fresh myrrh; apply it on her navel and place a bandage from cloth dipped in myrrh on it.

Case Ebers 793: 94,3-94,5
Another: dried human feces, mix with incense, fumigate the woman with it, and let the smoke enter inside her vagina.

Case Ebers 794: 94,5-94,7
Another: dried human feces, beer foam, rub the fingers of the woman with it. You should put it on all her limbs that hurt.

Case Ebers 795: 94,7-94,8
Another (remedy) for causing the uterus to leave into its place: ibis of wax, place (it) on the coals and let the smoke enter her vagina.

Case Ebers 796: 94,8-94,10
Determining good milk: when its smell is like crushed earth almonds. It is a way to determine.

Case Ebers 797: 94,10-94,11
Another (remedy) for causing a woman to give on the ground:
the plant *niaia*, have the woman sit on it to release.

Case Ebers 798: 94,11-94,13
Another (remedy) for causing everything that is in a woman's belly to come out:
sherds of a new vessel *hin*, grind with oil, heat, and pour into her vagina.

Case Ebers 799: 94,13-94,14
Another: mashed dates, salt from the Delta, oil, boil and drink at the temperature of a finger.

Case Ebers 800: 94,14-94,15
Another (remedy) for releasing the child from the belly of a woman:

salt from the Delta 1, white emmer 1, female rush 1; apply it on the bottom of her belly.

Case Ebers 801: 94,15-94,16
Another: fresh trigonella 1, honey 1; strain and drink for one day.

Case Ebers 802: 94,16-94,17
Another: fennel 1, incense 1, resin 1, *djesret* beer 1, fresh trigonella 1, fly droppings 1; make a suppository of it and place it in her womb.

Case Ebers 803: 94,17-94,18
Another: incense 1, oil 1; grease her belly with it.

Case Ebers 804: 94,18-94,19
Another: the plant *niaia* 1, mineral *kesenty* 1, wine 1; strain and drink for four days.

Case Ebers 805: 94,19
Another: *ished* fruits 1, *djesret* beer 1; pour into her vagina.

Case Ebers 806: 94,19-94,21
Another: fruits of the juniper 1, the plant *niaia* 1, cedar resin 1; make a suppository of it and place it in her vagina.

Case Ebers 807: 94,21-94,22
Another: turtle part *nis* 1, *hekun* beetles 1, cedar oil 1, *djesret* beer 1, oil 1; grind into one and apply on her.

Case Ebers 808: 95,1-95,3
The beginning of a remedy for not having the nipples go down:
bathe them in the blood of one whose menstruation has come for the first time. Rub it on her belly and both of her thighs so that *gesu* do not appear with her.

Case Ebers 809: 95,3-95,5
Another (remedy) for not having *gesu* with a woman:
dried swallow liver, grate with a fermented herb decoction. Apply it on the woman's breasts, on her belly, and on all of her limbs if *gesu* has appeared.

Case Ebers 810: 95,5–95,7
Another remedy for a breast that aches:
hetem mineral 1, bull bile 1, fly droppings 1, ochre 1; mix together and spread it on the breast for four days.

Case Ebers 811: 95,7–95,14
Enchantment for the breast:
It is the breast that hurt Isis in the swamps of Akhbity when she bore Shu and Tefnut. What to do for them (= both breasts): enchant them with sedge, with *seneb* grass seeds, with rush shoots, and with fibers from its inside, brought to drive away the (harmful) activities of the dead (male) and dead (female). **Incantation.**

Roll (it up) to the left, put it in a place of the dead (male) and dead (female). Do not urinate, do not bite, do not bleed, watch that opacity does not appear against people.

Recite the words over the sedge, *seneb* grass seeds, rush shoots, fibers from the top of its inside, roll to the left and make seven knots on it. Give it to her.

Case Ebers 812: 95,15–95,16
A remedy for driving away slime from the uterus:
dried myrtle leaves and the dregs of excellent beer; apply on her pelvis and her pubic region.

Case Ebers 813: 95,16–95,18
Another (remedy) for eating in her uterus and the occurrence of ulcers in her vagina:
fresh dates 1, leaves of the cinnamon tree 1, stone from the riverbank; grate in water, leave overnight (exposed) to the dew, and pour into her vagina.

Case Ebers 814: 95,18–95,19
Another: fresh dates 1, brain of a pig 1, *kesenty* mineral 1; immerse, leave overnight (exposed) to the dew, and pour into her vagina.

Case Ebers 815: 95,19–95,21
Another doing against great pain and suffering:
boiled cow milk 1, acacia leaves 1, *kesenty* mineral 1; grind together, leave overnight (exposed) to the dew, and pour into her vagina. It is (a remedy for) cooling.

Case Ebers 816: 95,21–95,22

Another: fresh dates 1, white oil 1, acacia leaves 1, oil 1, water; the same.

Case Ebers 817: 95,22–96,2

Another (remedy) for the occurrence of pains in the mouth of her vagina:

resin 1, ochre 1, *nehdet* mineral 1, incense 1, acacia leaves 1, spinal cord of a bull 1, *heny-ta* 1, water 1; mix together and pour into her vagina.

Case Ebers 818: 96,2–96,4

Another (remedy) for *kemit* in the uterus and the occurrence of ulcers in her vagina:

wild carrot 1 grate in water, incense 1, *kesenty* mineral 1; pour (it) into her vagina.

Case Ebers 819: 96,4–96,5

Another: earth almonds 1/8, fresh dates 1/8, acacia leaves 1/8, *kesenty* mineral 1/32, water 1/64 (grain measure), milk of asses; leave overnight (exposed to) the dew and pour into her vagina.

Case Ebers 820: 96,5–96,7

Another (remedy) for cooling the uterus and driving away its heat:

ground sorghum, nut grass; grind with oil and pour into her vagina. It is contraction of the uterus.

Case Ebers 821: 96,7–96,8

Another: grind hemp with honey and pour into her vagina. It is contraction (of the uterus).

Case Ebers 822: 96,8–96,9

Another: incense, celery; grind with cow milk, strain through a cloth, and pour into her vagina. It is contraction (of the uterus).

Case Ebers 823: 96,9–96,11

Another (remedy) for contraction of the uterus: wild carrot 1, honey 1, carob juice 1, milk 1; strain and have (it) poured into her vagina.

Case Ebers 824: 96,11

Another: *mesta* drink, pour (it) into her vagina.

Case Ebers 825: 96,11–96,12
Another: potamogeton juice, pour (it) into her vagina.

Case Ebers 826: 96,12
Another: *ketket* juice, pour (it) into her vagina.

Case Ebers 827: 96,12
Another: *niaia* juice, pour (it) into her vagina.

Case Ebers 828: 96,13–96,14
A remedy for getting out blood from a woman:
onion 1, wine 1; mix together and pour into her vagina.

Case Ebers 829: 96,14–96,15
Another: acacia leaves 1, moringa oil 1, oil 1, *pakh-seryt* plant 1, pea 1, honey 1; pour (it) into her vagina.

Case Ebers 830: 96,15–96,16
Another: fennel 1/8, honey 1/8, milk fat **a half of 1/64** (grain measure), sweet beer **1/64** (grain measure); pour (it) into her vagina for four days.

Case Ebers 831: 96,16–96,19
When you examine a woman from whom something like water and in the end like coagulated blood comes out.
    You should say of it: it is a scratch in her uterus.
    You should prepare for it: Nile mud from a pump, grate with honey and galenite, spread on a piece of cloth, and place (it) in her vagina for four days.

Case Ebers 832: 96,20–97,1
When you examine a woman whom one side of her pubic region hurts.
    You should say of it: it is an irregularity of her bleeding after it started.
    You should prepare for it: mashed onion, muskmelon, cedar sawdust; bandage her pubic region with it.

Case Ebers 833: 97,1–97,7
When you examine a woman with whom many years have passed without her bleeding coming. She vomits something like *hebebet*-water; her belly is like one afflicted with fever; it stops after she vomits.
    You should say of it: it is accumulation of the blood in her uterus due to

an enchantment [. . .] coitus. **You should prepare for her:** juniper fruits 1/32, cumin 1/64, incense 1/64, earth almonds 1/16; you should place cow milk 1/4 (grain measure) on the fire with bone marrow, add (the ingredients) to the milk, and drink for four days.

Case Ebers 834: 97,7–97,8
Another preparation for cutting pain (caused) by heat in the uterus:
brain of a bull 1, *kesenty* mineral 1, oil 1; mix together and pour into the vagina.

Case Ebers 835: 97,8–97,9
Another doing against the appearance of the disease *idju*:
shena, dried *khenesh*; grind and give it to him.

Case Ebers 836: 97,10–97,11
Restoring milk for a wet nurse who cares for a child:
the spine of the Nile bass, boil with oil and spread it on her back.

Case Ebers 837: 97,11–97,12
Another: barley sourdough, prepared on a fire with *khesau* plant. (To be) eaten by the woman whose legs are weakened.

Case Ebers 838: 97,13–97,14
Another **determination of a child on the day it is born:**
if he says "ny," he will live,
if he says "embi," he will die.

Case Ebers 839: 97,14–97,15
Another determination:
if his voice is wailing, he will die,
if he turns his face downward, he will die.

London Papyrus (BM 10059)
Case London 40: 13,9–13,14
[. . .] back [. . .] back, you who come! Back. [. . .] The gods who are at the head of Iunu (= Heliopolis) have been turned back. Do not fear, boy, I have brought you the best yarn, feathers of the black swallow, hairs of a fair ass, and the liver of a turtle. Recite what I have told you. Entry of those who come into (him) and come out of him.

This incantation (should be) recited above the best yarn, feathers of the black swallow, hairs of a fair ass, and the liver of a turtle, [a bundle rolled] to the left on which four knots have been made. Grease with pig liver and put it in the woman's rectum to turn away all blood and all enchantments. It is also (a preparation for) strengthening the egg and against dreaming. This incantation is recited over each knot.

Case London 41: 13,14–14,1

Another (method) for turning away bleeding:

Anubis came forth to prevent the flood from entering the pure territory of (the goddess) Tayet and thus to protect what is in her.

This incantation is recited over linen yarn on which a knot has been made. Place inside her vagina.

Case London 42: 14,1–14,2

Turning away the harmful activity of the dead or a god with the incantation:

Anubis, the flood is approaching the edge of the territory of (the goddess) Tayet. Get rid of what is in her!

Recite the words when you have placed two knots on linen yarn into the mouth of the inside of her vagina to turn away what has been (performed) against her.

Case London 45: 14,5–14,8

Enchanting the womb:

You . . . who have darkened for her, stretch this womb, descend to (your) place, and make your horn high. Raise your horn like Sekhathor. Horn against horn, shoulder against shoulder. The bowels of the rectum and belly have been as if [bound] since the time that what is has existed, because of the coming of the flood inside to close the mouth of the womb as Lower Egypt is closed in south Djadja, and as a mouth of a valley is closed.

Give [. . .] wound to the left.

Papyrus Carlsberg VIII

Case Carlsberg VIII 1: 1,1–1,3

[. . .] for assuming conception [. . .] all things [. . .] once.

You should prepare for her [assuming] conception. If not [. . .]

Case Carlsberg VIII 2: 1,3–1,5

[. . .] into fabric bags [. . .] sand from the coastline in the way [. . .] on them every day after they have been filled [. . .] dates. If it shows worms [. . .] she will not give birth. [. . .] worms, the born one will live. If [. . .]

Case Carlsberg VIII 3: 1,6–1,9

[. . .] you should [put] barley and emmer into a fabric bag [. . .] on it every day. [. . .] dates [. . .] she will give birth to a son [. . .] both together, she will give birth many times [. . .] If they do not [. . .]

Case Carlsberg VIII 4: 1,10–1,16

[. . .] woman not [. . .] You should place for the night a tuber of onion [. . .] [into] her vagina until the break of day.

If a stench appears in her mouth, she will give birth.

If [. . .] [she will] never [give birth].

Case Carlsberg VIII 5: 1,16–2,1

Another (way) to know one who will give birth from one who will not give birth:

you should fumigate her with [. . .] her vagina.

If she vomits from her mouth for feeling sick, she will never give birth.

If she has flatulence, [. . .] she will give birth.

Case Carlsberg VIII 6: 2,1–2,3

Another (way) to know one who will give birth [. . .]:

you should have the woman stand up at a jamb of the door in [. . .] and you should look into her eyes.

If you see [. . .] the other like a Nubian, she will never give birth.

If [. . .] in one color, she will give birth.

Case Carlsberg VIII 7: 2,3–2,6

[. . .] from one who will not give birth. You should make her drink up [. . .] fresh dates 1/64 (grain measure), dates [. . .] mashed dates 1/8, wine [. . .]

[. . .] feeling sick, she will never give birth.

[. . .], she will give birth.

Papyrus Berlin 3038

Case Berlin 13: 1,11–2,1

[. . . . . .] honey, thyme [. . .] breast (to) drive away pain.

Case Berlin 14: 2,1–2,2

A remedy to drive away swelling in the breast and all the limbs:
a grain of white emmer, a powder from carob, a powder from dates, natron, sourdough from dates; grind finely, mix together, and apply on them.

Case Berlin 15: 2,2–2,3

Another: powder from carob, honey, and (mineral) great protection, grind; the same.

Case Berlin 16: 2,3

Another: powder from the *tjun*-herb, salt from the Delta, fresh *ihu*-plant, honey; the same.

Case Berlin 17: 2,3–2,4 = Case Ebers 810: 95,5–95,7

A remedy for a breast that aches:
bile of a bull, fly droppings, ochre; mix together and spread on the breast.

Case Berlin 18: 2,4–2,5

A remedy made when a breast aches:
natron, salt; boil with honey and carob and thoroughly spread on the breast.

Case Berlin 30: 3,5–3,6

Another (remedy) for driving away cough in a child:
dried dates, grind finely with a *hin* of milk; to be drunk by the child.

Case Berlin 192: verso 1,1–1,2

[. . .] a woman without having conceived:
fumigate her with sorghum in her womb so she does allow acceptance [. . .]
[. . . You make] a remedy for her to release it: oil 1/64 (grain measure), celery 1/64 (grain measure), sweet beer 1/64 (grain measure); boil and drink for four mornings.

Case Berlin 193: 1,3–1,4

[. . .] a woman who will give birth and a woman who will not give birth:
watermelon ground and pressed with the milk of one who has given birth to a boy, prepared as a drink-remedy and (to be) swallowed by the woman. If she vomits, she will give birth. If she has flatulence, she will never give birth.

Case Berlin 194: 1,5–1,6

What is said of it as another remedy:

watermelon pressed with the milk of one who has given birth to a boy, pour (it) into her womb. If she vomits, she will give birth. If she has flatulence, she will never give birth.

Case Berlin 195: 1,7–1,8

Another determination of a woman who will not give birth: [. . .] things [. . .] you should fumigate her with hippopotamus dung.

If [. . .] urine along with feces or has flatulence at the same time, she will give birth. If not, she will not give birth, as she is one for whom all things stand.

Case Berlin 196: 1,9–1,11

Another determination: when she lies down, spread fresh oil on her bosom, both of her arms, and her shoulders. Get up early in the morning to see her.

If you find her veins green and nice, not sunken, the birth will be calm. If you find them sunken and like the color of her body, it is unhealthy (?).

If you find them green and dark when you see her, she will give birth later.

Case Berlin 197: 1,11–1,13

Another determination: you should take her fingers into your palm, bend her arm, and move it over her body. Then grasp her forearm in your fingers and palpate on the worms (= veins) on all sides of her arm.

If the veins in her arms pulsate against your hand, you should say: she will be pregnant.

Case Berlin 198: 2,1–2,2

Another determination: have her stand up in the jamb of the door.

If you find the look of her eyes one like an Asian and the other like a Nubian, she will not give birth.

If you find them in one color, she will give birth.

Case Berlin 199: 2,2–2,4

Another determination (whether) a woman will give birth or will not give birth:

barley and emmer; the woman (should) water (them) with her urine every day, like dates and like sand in two bags.

If they all survive, she will give birth.

If barley survives, it is a boy.
If emmer survives, it is a girl.
If they do not survive, she will not give birth.

Book for Mother and Child (Papyrus Berlin 3027)

Case *Book for Mother and Child* A: 1,1–1,4

[. . .] a green bead from malachite is on it, a red bead from jasper is on it, the beads have fallen on . . . into water, on the scales of fish in the river, on the feathers of birds in the heavens. Flow out, disease *neshu*, descend on the earth!

This incantation is recited above three beads, one of lapis lazuli, another of jasper, another of malachite, hung on the best yarn, and placed on the neck of the child.

Case *Book for Mother and Child* B: 1,4–1,9

Another: Flow out, disease *temyt*, bonebreaker, stone tearer, entering [. . .] the blood vessels, go out into the swamps, to the swamps, to the fields, to the fields, all the way to the end of the vegetation. The voice of Ra calls Nephthys, because the stomach of this [child] whom Isis bore hurts. What is he to be enchanted with? He is to be enchanted with *itenu en h* [. . .] for the (disease) to fall and go out. Behold, [fire] has been created. What is it to be extinguished with? It is to be extinguished with *itenu en h* [. . .] *itenu en h* will [. . .] it for it (to be) driven away from the head, from the top of the head, and from all of the limbs that Khnum has created for this child born to his mother.

Case *Book for Mother and Child* C: 1,9–2,6

Another: Flow out, you (male) who come in the dark, who crawl with your nose behind you, with face turned, whom it escapes why he has come.

Flow out, you (female) who come in the dark, who crawl with your nose behind you, with face turned, whom it escapes why she has come.

Have you come to kiss this child? I will not allow you to kiss him. Have you come to his comfort? I will not allow you to give him comfort. Have you come to hurt him? I will not allow you to hurt him. Have you come to take him away? I will not allow you to take him away. I have prepared his protection (= amulet) of yellow sweet clover, which does you harm; onion, which ruins you; honey; sweet for people but bitter for those who are dead; from *sedeb* (tail of the sacred) fish *abedju*, from a piece of cloth, and from the spine of the Nile bass.

Case *Book for Mother and Child* D: 2,6–2,10

An incantation [against] enemies . . .

You (female) who are busy making bricks for your father Osiris! You who have spoken against your father Osiris! He lives from the plant *djais* and honey. Flow out, Asian, who comes from the mountains, Nubian, who comes from the desert. Are you a servant? Hence, come out by vomiting. Are you noble? Hence, come out in his urine, come out in the mucus of his nose, come out in the sweat of his limbs! My hands rest on this child and the hands of Isis rest on him, as she laid her hands on her own son Horus.

Case *Book for Mother and Child* E: 2,10–5,7

Driving away the disease *neshu* from all of the limbs of a child.

You are Horus! Wake up as Horus! You are the living Horus! I am driving away the disease that is in your body and the torment that is in your limbs like a crocodile quick in the middle of the river and a snake of fast poison. Knife in the hands of a bold butcher, do not feed on its limbs, do not enter its marrow, watch your plows, their pots will be broken, their knives (will be made blunt). Flow out, disease *neshu*, come down! Pus, brother of blood, friend of discharges, father of swellings! Jackal from the south, come to sleep and come to the place where your beautiful (females) are, who have rubbed myrrh in their hair and fresh incense on their shoulders. Flow out, disease *neshu*, come down!

Do not affect his head, avoid spilling over it! Do not affect the crown of his head, avoid defecating on it! Do not affect his forehead, avoid warping it! Do not affect his eyebrows, avoid making them fall out! Do not affect his eyes, avoid eye ailments, avoid amblyopia! Do not affect his nose, avoid nose maladies! Do not affect his breasts, it is mandrake of Hathor! Do not affect his mouth, avoid secrets! Do not affect his vertebrae, avoid breakage! Do not affect his throat, avoid decay! Do not affect his tongue, because it is a snake from the mouth of a cave! Do not affect his lips, avoid *maa*! Do not affect his chin, because it is a duck's tail! Do not affect his temples, avoid deafness! Do not affect his ears, avoid hearing loss! Do not affect his neck, avoid constriction! Do not affect his shoulders, they are live falcons! Do not affect his arms, avoid . . . ! Do not affect his fingers, avoid . . . ! Do not affect his bosom, avoid making it falling! Do not affect his breasts, they are the breasts of Hathor! Do not affect his skin, avoid damage! Do not affect his stomach, it is Nut born by gods! Do not affect his [. . .], avoid union! Do not affect his navel, it is a solitary (= morning) star! Do not affect his pubic region, avoid what the gods forbade to the born! Do not affect his penis, avoid chafing! Do not affect his pelvis, avoid bad odor! Do not affect his back, avoid [. . .] it! Do not affect his loins; it is the spirit of the son of Sekhmet! Do not affect his rectum, avoid hemorrhoids! Do not affect his buttocks, they are ostrich eggs! Do not affect his thighs, avoid driving them away! Do not affect his knee, avoid paralysis! Do not affect his ankles, avoid the upper leg!

Flow out, disease *neshu*, come down, be spat out under the soles of its feet [. . .] Geb, the most fertile of the gods. Flood has come to the house of the disease *neshu*, cloth on its shoulders for its inhabitants [and said] to this Asian (female). Are you coming, you Asian? Are you entering, you Asian? I had come to request spitting out when I found that you were sitting happily with your . . . in your hand that which says [. . .] form for [. . .] dough [. . .] . . . foods of the disease *neshu* on the twigs of the bryony, on the bolls of the *sar* plant, on the twigs of the sycamore, on the creator of the north breeze. Flow out, disease *neshu*, come out onto the ground!

Case *Book for Mother and Child* F: 5,8–6,8

[Incantation for separating] this [child from] the body of this [woman].

Meskhenet, you have [a soul], spirit, and all that is necessary. Meskhenet, (created) by the hand of Atum, born to Shu and Tefnut. A child is coming! It is known to you, in your name Meskhenet, how to make the spirit for this child that is in the body of this woman. I have prepared for him a royal order for Geb to make for him the soul and spirit and all that is necessary, Nut (to prepare) diapers for the children of this woman. Do not allow any evil thing to be uttered, because you are good. Do not injure the right by the evil mouth. Satisfied! Drive it from him . . . Nut, you have taken (to yourself) all of the gods, and their lights are stars. They have not abandoned their stars. Their protection comes so that I can protect this woman. [**This incantation] is recited over two bricks on which** [a woman gives birth . . .] bird [. . .] and incense into the fire.

Do this enchanting shrouded in a diaper of fine linen and have in your hand a staff of [. . .]

Case *Book for Mother and Child* G: 6,8–7,1

Another: I was begotten at a sacred place, born in the water canal of the gods, and washed in the lake of the kings. My things are for you, my things are inside [. . .]

Recite the words against [. . . . . .], for the child to be brought (to the world) without anything evil. Good!

Case *Book for Mother and Child* H: 7,1–7,3
Expulsion of *baa*:
   tepaut of a sycamore, fresh dates, a *hemu* part of the castor oil plant, hemp, fibers of the plant *debyt*, the *mesta* drink; (to be) drunk by the woman.

Case *Book for Mother and Child* I: 7,3–7,5
Another: bolls of papyrus plant, earth almonds; grind and mix with the milk of one who has given birth to a boy. Give a *hin* to this child for him to survive the day and night and for his healthy sleep.

Case *Book for Mother and Child* K: 7,5–7,6
Another: twigs of the *nebu*-plant; mash with water in a *hin*-vessel. Give it to him to drink up.

Case *Book for Mother and Child* L: 7,6–8,3
Driving away *sesemy*:
   Oh you who are in water, hurry and tell this judge who is in his temple, Sekhmet, who comes to see him, the Musician (= Hathor) who rises, Wadjet, Lady of Buto: Bring her this milk. You Great One, who are in your cave, make for her six celebrations (of festival) *denit* (= the first quarter of the moon), twice in Iunu (= Heliopolis). Let the Great One give an eye for the eye that has seen Seth.
   Recite [. . . when] giving the child, or your *(sic)* mother, a cooked mouse **to eat.** Put its bones on his neck in a sachet of fine cloth tied with seven knots.

Case *Book for Mother and Child* M: 8,3–9,3
Medicine for placing hands on the child.
   A voice strong and great, which tamarix . . . its territory with a cobra that came from the West when it found the path, Iaret. Anubis, you have come from Djedu (= Busiris).
   You who do not eat the fish *adju*, avoid your rolls of fabric being . . . You who do not eat the fish *adju*, avoid your tombs being robbed. You who do not eat the fish *adju*, [avoid] your funerary equipment being taken away. You who do not eat the fish *adju*, avoid the offerings presented [to you] being carried away.
   You have eaten the fish *adju*, sipped its part, decorated yourself with a limb from it. You know what is up; you know what is down. You have eaten the whole fish *adju*, theft is bad.
   Incantations (for) person N, (born to) a woman.

Make from a part . . . of the fish *adju*, make one knot on that and put it on the neck.

Case *Book for Mother and Child* N: 9,3–9,7

Hathor, you who are in the north sky and whose . . . have united with . . . hair of Itery with . . .

I have divided the time of union, I have found time for my hair (?), I have set a time and place (?) like hair (?) . . . complete. Twice!

Strong body, boy, [. . .] you have come to Hathor to give the dead an incantation that causes bitterness. The child is warm [. . .] under [my hand and my] fingers. [Protection] for protection, protection (= amulet) comes. Make a **braid from hair, tie four knots (on it), and put it on the neck of the child.**

Case *Book for Mother and Child* O: 9,7–2,2

An amulet for a woman who has milk.

Lamentation to the skies and screams (from labor pain) to Duat. Distress in [. . .] I put [. . .] my hands [. . .] on them [. . .] to procure a channel that is empty, which does not have any fish. Sobek has eaten the offering (?) [. . .], which are in it. Ra has been turned to his side, twice. She said: make justice for what was done by that enemy, the dead (male) and the dead (female), as an enchantment against milk. It has the diseases *baa*, my arms are inverse, the breasts are in the hand of Tayet. Go out, you who hear, seek [. . .] his bread. You wind it [. . .] then you weave it, then [you wrap] it on the thigh, you bind it into three knots until it is bound, and put it on the neck of Horus when he awakes, so that he could free himself from his enemy.

It is made from four linen threads from [. . .] they are wound, woven, and also wrapped. Tie four knots in it and put it on the neck of the child, so that it would free itself from its enemy.

Case *Book for Mother and Child* P: 2,2–2,7

Incantation on knots for a child and a nestling.

Are you warm in the nest? Are you hot in the thicket? Your mother is not with you, no sister is there to help (you), no wet nurse is there to provide protection (to you). Let someone bring a ball of gold, a grain of garnet, a small seal, a crocodile, a hand to drive away Ta-merut, to warm up [your] limbs, to defeat this enemy (male) and this enemy (female) from the West. Come out, you protection!

This incantation is recited above small balls of gold, grains of garnet, a small seal, a crocodile, and a hand, which are strung on a fine thread, making an amulet to be put on the neck of the child. Good!

Case *Book for Mother and Child* Q: 2,7–3,3
Incantation that is read aloud over a child in the early morning.

You are coming out, Ra, you are coming out. When you saw this dead (male) coming toward N, born of N, (along with) the dead (female) to offend her when she is doing what is necessary to not let her child be taken from her hand. Protect me, Ra, my lord. I will not give you; I will not give the child when there are evil powers in this child (?). My hand is resting on her, the small seal is your protection. Look, I am protecting you.

This incantation is to be recited above the small seal and hand that made the amulet, bind it into seven knots, (namely) a knot in the morning, another in the evening, nicely until seven knots are completed.

Case *Book for Mother and Child* R: 3,3–3,7
You are coming out, Ra, and setting there. When you saw the dead (male) coming toward N, born of N, (along with) the dead (female) to offend her when she is doing what is necessary to not let her (child) be taken from her hand. Protect me, my lord Ra, says (mother N). I will not give you; I do not give my burden to a thief, male or female. I am placing my hand on you; the small seal is your protection. Ra is setting; look, I am protecting you.

This incantation is to be recited in the evening when Ra is setting.

Case *Book for Mother and Child* S: 3,8–4,2
An amulet for safeguarding the body, which is delivered over a child when the light rises.

You are rising, Ra, you are rising. When you saw this dead (male) coming toward her, N, born of N, [along with the dead (female)] to offend her when she is doing what is necessary, (then) do not let him/her take her son in his/her arms. Protect me, my lord Ra, says N, born of N. I will not give you; I will not give my burden to a thief, male or female, from the West. My hand is resting on you, my small seal is your protection, says Ra when he rises. Come out, protection!

Case *Book for Mother and Child* T: 4,2–4,6
What to recite when Ra is setting.

You are setting, Ra, you are setting. When you saw this dead (man) coming toward her, N, born of N, (along with) the dead (female), to offend her when she is doing what is necessary to not let her burden be taken from her hand. Protect me, my lord Ra, says N, born of N. I will not give you; I do not give [my] burden to a thief, male or female, from the West. My hand is resting on you, my small seal is [your] protection, says Ra when he is setting. Come out, protection!

An amulet made for this child.

Your protection is the protection of the heavens and the protection of the land; your protection is the protection of the night; your protection is the protection of the day; your protection is the protection of gold; your protection is the protection of agate; your protection is the protection of Ra; your protection is the protection of those seven gods who kissed the earth and destroyed those who steal hearts from their places.

The crown of your head is like that of Ra, healthy child. Look, the back of your head is like Osiris's; your forehead is like that of Satis, lady of Abu (= Elephantine); your lungs (hair) are like Neith's; your eyebrows are like those of the Lady of the East; your eyes are like those of the Lord of All; your nose is like the herald of the gods; your ears are like two Iaret (= cobras); your shoulder is like that of a live falcon; your arm is like Horus's and the other like Seth's; your hip is like that of Sopdu (= Sirius) and the other like that of Nut, the parent of the gods, the sanctuary that is born by the pure place in Iunu (= Heliopolis) and in which all the gods are. Your heart *ib* is like Montu's; your heart *haty* is like Atum's; your lungs are like Min's; your gall bladder is like Nefertem's; your spleen is like Sobek's; your liver is like [that of Lord Henennisut]; your stomach is in health; your navel is like [that] of the Solitary (= Morning Star); your thigh is like Isis's and the other like Nephthys's; your feet are like [. . .] they carry [. . .]; your ankles are two vessels from which a river rises; your [toes] are baby snakes [. . .]; enchanting [. . .] enchant in your name.

There is no limb on you empty of [divine], every god says protecting your name [. . .] all milk that you drink and that is in her, every armful into which you are placed, every thigh on which you are placed, the clothes in which you are dressed, all [. . .] in which you live, every protection that is done for you, every refuge into which you are given, the knot (protection) for you, every amulet that is put on your neck.

Through them he protects you, through them he makes you healthy, through them he heals you, through them he reconciles all the gods and all the goddesses for you.

Incantation for a woman when she is bleeding and birth has begun.

Be you praised, . . . you Isis spinning and you Nephthys tying divine threads into seven knots for you to be protected by them, you healthy child, N, son of N, to become healthy, to be healed, so that all of the gods and all of

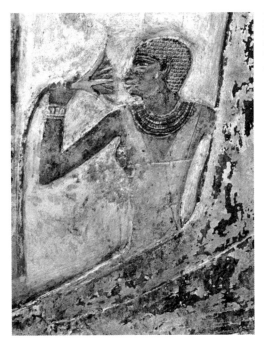

Fig. 37. Merut, the wife of Judge Inti, kneels at the feet of her spouse and smells a lotus flower. (Sixth Dynasty, tomb of Inti at Abusir, photo: K. Voděra)

the goddesses would be reconciled for you, so that the stealing male enemy would be struck dead, so that the stealing female enemy would be defeated, so that the names *(sic)* of those that denigrate you would be closed, as the mouths were closed and the mouths were sealed of seventy-seven asses when they were in the Lake of Two Knives. I know them and I know their names; they are unknown to the one who is planning to harm this child to become ill.

Incantation: **this incantation is recited [. . .] four times over the seven balls of agate, seven of gold, seven linen threads that have been woven by two mothers, of whom one wove them and the other wound them. An amulet with seven knots on it will be made and put around the neck of the child (to provide) protection for [his] body.**

Medicine and Women

In ancient Egyptian society, a woman enjoyed a respectable position and was especially revered in marriage as a wife and mother (Strouhal 2002, 51–61; Vachala 2007b, 435–51). Depictions in Egyptian tombs capture the immense charm of Egyptian girls, women, and mothers. The female body is at the same time shown without shame, the breasts of women are often revealed, and young girls are sometimes entirely nude but for lumbar belts and jewelry.

Women's problems are dealt with in a great number of the cases described in medical texts. It is not surprising, because women's predestination to bear offspring brought with it great attention from the entire society and frequently also the risk of complications. Neither the Kahun Papyrus nor any of the other papyri with prescriptions concerning women contains treatment by surgical operations, whether in women's illnesses or in childbirth, for example the wedging of the fetus in the descent through the birth canal. On the other hand, giving birth was considered a common part of a woman's life. Girls were married after reaching puberty, whose sign was the first menstruation, and they soon afterward began to give birth. They often had children every three years (or even more often), and therefore it was not a rarity to find five to ten children in a family, despite the high neonatal and infant mortality. The average lifespan of the common people was between twenty and twenty-five years; with the aristocracy and rich people, who could afford to be mummified, between thirty and thirty-five years. As a result of this, the generations came and went quickly.

It seems that the medical care of women in ancient Egypt was the exclusive domain of women, largely nameless, likely older, experienced birth assistants. The presence of midwives is proved on many reliefs and depictions, but it is not clear whether they were specialized midwives who made their living with this activity and were called to various households for childbirths. In the written documents, we do not find any expressions that would clearly label the profession of midwives in the Egyptian language, although some experts propose that women labeled as "servants of Heqet" (the goddess connected with births, fig. 38; Nunn 1996, 102) could have assisted at childbirths. No evidence of their activities has been preserved, however, and it is more likely that the role of midwives was filled by experienced women from the family and milieu of the expectant mother. The depictions or descriptions of births that we find on temple reliefs usually capture the moment of the birth of a god or king, where goddesses appeared in the role of birth assistants (fig. 39). The only preserved written description is a tale from the Westcar Papyrus (Berlin 3033; Erman 1890), where Rudjdjedet, the wife of the high priest of the supreme sun god Ra, gives birth to triplets, the future kings. It is a magical birth, in which the mother in childbed is helped by the goddesses Isis, Nephthys, Heqet, and Meskhenet. Isis and Nephthys supported the mother, Heqet accelerated the birth, and Meskhenet declared the newborn children as the future kings (Simpson 2003, 21–22).

The expectant mother, whether of royal or common origin, was identified with the goddess Isis. This idea refers to the ancient myth of the birth of the god

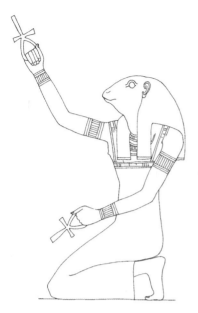

Fig. 38. The goddess Heqet, in the form of a woman with a frog's head, was connected with motherhood and birth, but also with rebirth. (Eighteenth Dynasty, Hatshepsut Temple at Deir al-Bahari, drawing: J. Malátková after Naville 1896, pl. XLVIII)

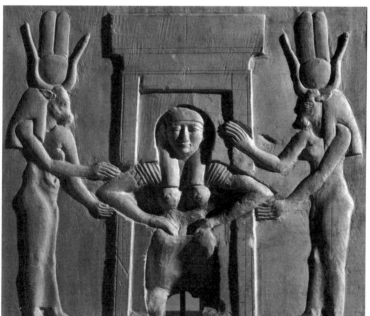

Fig. 39. In childbirth, which took place in a squatting position, the mother is supported from both sides by the goddess Hathor, depicted with a cow's head and a sun disc between the horns. (Ptolemaic Period, Egyptian Museum, Cairo [CG 40627], photo: M. Zemina)

Horus, legendary heir to the Egyptian throne. According to the myth, Horus's father, the god Osiris, was murdered by his own brother Seth, who seized rule over the Two Lands (unified Egypt). Osiris's wife Isis, well versed in magic, for a short time revived her husband magically and conceived a son with him (fig. 40). Then she hid in the bushes of the Nile Delta in Akhbity (in Greek Khemmis) and in this hiding place gave birth to Osiris's son and heir Horus. Thanks to her magical powers, she always managed to protect Horus from the danger and intrigues of the treacherous Seth until Horus came of age and ruled over Egypt. While she was in hiding, Isis was assisted by a great number of other gods, primarily her sister Nephthys, the jackal god Anubis, and so on (Wilkinson 2003, 146–49). The period of childbirth was perceived as a critical moment for the activity of magical powers, and many of the methods described in the texts also include magical incantations referring to Isis and Horus and other gods and goddesses, who were to assure protection of both the expectant mother and the newborn. These were the conditions under which common cases of births and postnatal care were apparently resolved.

For more complicated cases of a gynecological nature, physicians were likely called. Specialized physicians for women's problems are not specifically

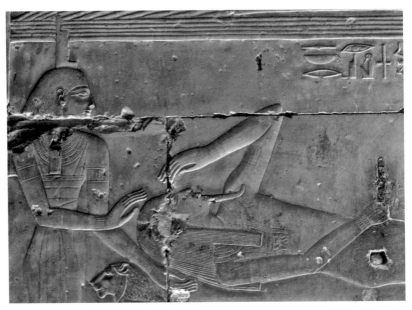

Fig. 40. By means of magic, the goddess Isis gently revives her dead husband Osiris, lying on a cot, to enable him to conceive their son Horus with her. (Nineteenth Dynasty, Temple of Seti I in Abydos, photo: M. Megahed)

identified in Egyptian documents, and we do not know of any term in the Egyptian language that would label a woman's doctor or obstetrician. In contrast, other professions were already specialized at the time of the Old Kingdom; for example, we know of physicians specializing in eye or gastroenterological disorders. Gynecology, however, was apparently one of the components of the work of common general practitioners, who were called to complicated births and other serious cases.

Whether the branch of women's medical science could have been performed by female physicians, so that the intimate problems of the gentle sex would remain hidden to unauthorized males, is not entirely proved. Of the many dozens of famous ancient Egyptian physicians, there are only a handful of women. Lady Overseer of the Lady Physicians Peseshet held her office in the Fifth–Sixth Dynasties and is so far the earliest known female doctor in history. Her funeral stele was placed in the tomb of the scribe Akhethotep, who seems to have been her son, in the famous cemetery in Giza (Hassan 1932, 81–84, fig. 143; Nunn 1996, 130). It is possible that the office of Peseshet was related to female physicians caring for the health of the queen mother within the royal palace (Robins 1993, 116).

Egyptian physicians were very well acquainted with the anatomy of female external sex organs; on the other hand, their ideas on the internal arrangement of the body were not always entirely precise. The Egyptians called the pubic region or genitals *kenes*; for the vulva (pudenda) or womb, we know the label *kat*. The vagina was called *shed* or *iuf*, which also meant 'meat.' The breast or bosom was labeled as *kabet* or *shena*, whereas the breast itself was *mendjet*. The uterus had the designation *idet*, and this expression could sometimes be used also in the wider sense of 'stomach.' The fetus in the body of the woman was sometimes described as *meset*, which is derived from the verb *mes*, 'to give birth,' but the fetus could also be called *wenu* or *suhet*, which literally means 'egg.' It is unlikely that Egyptians would have known the human egg and its function. The connection of the human fetus with the concept of an egg is, rather, related to the concept of the young as a small bird hatching from the mother's womb. This idea is also confirmed by many protective magical incantations that compare a child to a small bird.

The cases that we find recorded in the preserved texts can be divided by themes as well as by the methods of treating the problem, although there are also differences in the form and formulation. The cases described in more detail begin with a description of the symptoms and determination of the diagnosis. There then follows a prescription of the medicines of an herbal or animal origin. Such a format appears particularly in the first seventeen cases on the Kahun Papyrus and also on the Smith Papyrus, occasionally also on the Ebers Papyrus. The other cases are usually briefer, and the majority contain only the prescription with the ingredients of the remedy; some begin with the words "Another remedy for . . . " or merely "Another."

The topics of the cases include a wide range of problems, from pain of the hypogastrium and pain of the breasts, through cramps and bleeding, all the way to problems in urination. Cases for easing childbirth and resolving postnatal problems are also abundantly represented. An extensive group of cases deals with tests of female fertility in contrast to sterility and determining the due date for a birth or the sex of the unborn fetus. In addition, the methods for achieving conception, or on the other hand prescriptions for its prevention, hence natural contraceptive means, are recorded. Many women's problems were unclear for physicians, their symptoms were frequently interpreted mistakenly, and the treatment was often based on the application of preparations in connection with magical incantations. Surgical treatment, successful in many cases described in the previous chapter, was not applied in these cases, and this seems to be the reason that prognoses were also lacking.

Many times, the text has not been preserved in its entirety, because papyri in the course of the last three to four millennia have been torn, and today only their smaller or larger fragments are available. Some cases hence have gaps and often are hard to understand.

Pains

Pains are undoubtedly one of the most frequent signs of illness and also appear as the main manifestation, with a large number of cases devoted to women's problems, but the cause of the pains is rarely given in the texts, and it can be supposed that it was often unknown to ancient Egyptian healers.

The texts mention pains of various parts of the female body, including the eyes, teeth, neck, or limbs, and also refer to the connection between these pains and the womb. For us, however, the connection with gynecological illness in these cases is often entirely unclear. The symptoms connected with the womb could be interpreted with the hypothesis that the uterus, peculiar to women, was considered as the essence or symbol of women's difference from men.

Nevertheless, some of the problems described could be related to the pains that often accompany women's menstrual cycles. These complicating phenomena accompanying menstruation are usually the most distinctive from its beginning (premenstrual syndrome), with their peak in the middle of the menstrual bleeding, when they manifest themselves in the lower abdomen and back and can shoot even into the thighs (dysmenorrhea). They are sometimes

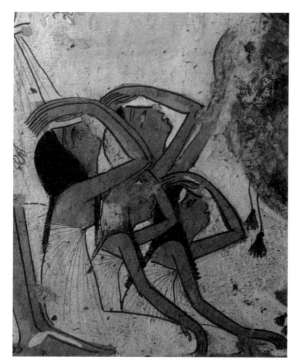

Fig. 41. The female mourners at a funeral weep copiously, and their gestures reflect their deep suffering over the death of the dignitary being buried. (Nineteenth Dynasty, tomb of Userhat [TT 51] in Sheikh Abd al-Qurna, photo: M. Zemina)

accompanied by vomiting, flatulence, breast tenderness, headaches, and neurological symptoms most often of the character of a migraine, discomfort, vomiting, and diarrhea. Moreover, in some women, transient mid-cycle pain occurs in the hypogastrium (intermenstrual pain), caused by irritation of the peritoneum by follicular fluid released during ovulation. Light bleeding can appear at the same time (Macků and Čech 2002, 79).

Other than these cyclically repeating problems, a woman could become ill from a great number of other painful conditions, primarily inflammations from mixed bacterial infections affecting various levels of her reproductive system—vulva (vulvitis), vagina (vaginitis), cervix (cervicitis), uterus (endometritis, myometritis, and perimetritis), fallopian tube (salpingitis), and fallopian tube with ovary (tubo-ovarian abscess). These are joined by various forms of tuberculosis, predominantly its female genital form (particularly tuberculous salpingitis), which is rare today but existed in ancient Egypt. Of the venereal diseases, gonorrhea and others could cause problems. On the other hand, lues (syphilis) and modern diseases like AIDS were not yet known among the ancient Egyptians.

In other cases, however, the pains described could be related to the abnormal position of the uterus, with accretions of the uterus and surrounding organs or with infections of the appendix (appendicitis). The uterus, which is firmly fixed in the lesser pelvis by connective tissues, was imagined by the ancient Egyptians as freely moving. They considered its movement or incorrect position in the abdominal cavity to be the cause or accompaniment of some disease symptoms.

Kahun 1: Pains of the eyes and neck
The case considers eye pains as a manifestation or consequence of the activity (which in Egyptian is called *khau*) of the uterus. This expression is sometimes interpreted as 'discharge,' but it is more likely a more general disorder of the function of the uterus, which could be accompanied by pains in various parts of a woman's body. In this case, fumigation of the eyes and also of the vulva is recommended. The patient was further to eat fresh (perhaps raw) donkey liver, which could have an invigorating effect with the quantity of vitamins and hematopoietic (erythropoietic or anti-anemic) factors.

Kahun 3: Pains of the pubic region, rectum, and inner sides of the thighs
The symptoms described in this case are here again considered as the manifestations *(khau)* of the uterus, but indicate rather problems of the evacuation of the rectum. The medicine is a mixture of 480 ml *(hin)* of cow's milk boiled with earth almonds and the seeds of *shasha* in equal amounts, which was to be drunk after cooling for four mornings. The drinking of this mixture on an empty stomach after waking up could actually be effective.

Kahun 7: Pains of the legs and feet after walking
Manifestations *(khau)* of the uterus also included pains in the upper and lower parts of the leg that occurred after a longer walk. For the cure, it was sufficient to smear the affected legs with mud. Leg pains when walking may emerge from a whole range of causes—swelling connected with the feelings of "heavy legs" is one of the symptoms of inflammation of the veins and thrombosis, swelling around the ankles signals cardiac insufficiency, swelling accompanies the injury of various parts of the leg, and so on. Pains in walking are not usually related to a disorder of an empty womb. However, when the uterus is enlarged during the third trimester of pregnancy by the developing fetus and amniotic fluid, swelling of the lower legs can occur as a consequence of vena caval compression impeding venous drainage from the large leg veins back to the heart.

Kahun 8: Pains of the nape, pubic region, and ears

If a woman has pain of the nape, ears (so that she does not hear), and pubic region, according to the text they are the fault of strong cramps *(neriu)* of the womb. The problem is to be resolved by removing impurities (detritus) from the uterus, namely the peeled mucous membrane or coagulated blood. It could be a symptom of dysmenorrhea with an accompanying migraine.

Kahun 9: Pain of the womb and limbs

The case describes pains of the womb and all of the limbs, which hurt as if beaten. The formulation expressing the diagnosis of the Egyptian physician has been only partially preserved, and Griffith (1898, 8) reads it as a "disorder of the womb" *(sau)*. In contrast, for example Nunn (1996, 197) considers the symptoms described as signs of rape. The text recommends treatment with oil, which the patient has to ingest.

Kahun 11: Strong cramps

A shaking woman bent from pain on a bed is troubled by a strong cramp or constriction *(amemu)* of the uterus. According to the text, it will be removed by drinking 960 ml (2 *hin*) of the drink *khawy* and vomiting it immediately. Cramping pains could appear, for instance, with a woman at the beginning of menstruation.

Kahun 12: Leg pain

Of a somewhat different character are isolated pains of the leg, originating, for example, as a consequence of muscle exhaustion, perhaps by long-term or difficult walking when carrying water or other burdens, which may or may not be connected with their swelling. According to this prescription, bandages soaked in myrrh should be applied on the painful legs of the woman, which might have had a cooling effect. The further text is preserved incompletely, and the gaps make the comprehension of the case more difficult. If the bandages do not help and movement continues to be painful, it is a more serious illness. The application of milk fat from fresh fat and myrrh is recommended.

Kahun 13: Pain of the leg and one side of the abdomen (?), tumor (?) of the womb

Pains of the leg and one side of the abdomen (?) are caused, according to the text, by a bending of the uterus called in Egyptian *kahu*. The patient receives a composite medicine composed of pine nuts, vitex, and a part of yellow nutsedge; she should then be laid to sleep so that the side that hurts is not burdened. The further text is interwoven with gaps, which make its comprehension much more difficult. The patient is to chew two medicines. When she has evacuated herself and done everything according to the advice, swelling may still remain. If the physician feels something solid in the uterus, it is a disease that was then incurable. This case could describe a tumor, in this case probably benign.

Kahun 16: Pains of the limbs and eye sockets

If all of the extremities and the eye sockets of a woman hurt, there is again, according to the Egyptian physician, a connection with female illness. According to the text, it is an illness *kemtu* of the womb, which can be treated with the listed prescription composed of oil, fruits of the *ished* and *iwehu*, flour, and pine nuts. In a ground and boiled state, the medicine was given for three days.

Ramesseum III.A II. 7–8: Leg pain

In this case, a woman is suffering from pains in the upper and lower parts of the legs. The diagnosis has unfortunately not been preserved, because the text is incomplete. The prescription is composed of mixtures prepared from the pulp of the pods of carob, muskmelon, and other ingredients, which have unfortunately not been preserved.

Kahun 5: Toothache *(tiau)*

This case describes strong pains of the teeth and gums, thus the periodontium. Even these manifestations were attributed to the uterus, perhaps because the Egyptians believed in the connection between the sexual and digestive tracts of a woman. Bardinet (1995, 222) on the other hand, connects cramps in the jaw with manifestations of tetanus; Westendorf (1999, 413) considers the described manifestations as strong cramps of the chewing apparatus. *Tiau* also appears in two additional cases in the same text, and Case Kahun 33 documents that pains of the teeth or cramps of the muscles of mastication described in this text could be connected with the pains that a woman experienced in childbirth. A woman suffering from these problems was to be treated by fumigation with oil, incense, and rinsing with ass urine. When this treatment was unsuccessful, when pains appeared in the woman's abdomen from the navel to the buttocks, it was an incurable disease. These pains could be caused by various things, one of which could be colic, as presumed by Griffith (1898, 7). Bardinet, however, considers a discharge as one of the possible interpretations, which nevertheless had no connection with pain of the teeth (Bardinet 1995, 222).

Kahun 24: Toothache *(tiau)*

This case contains another brief prescription for relieving a toothache, which includes a finely ground stem of a date palm (perhaps the ribs of the palm leaves) mixed with sweet beer. The suffering woman was to sit with her legs spread wide apart on this mixture. The effect of this treatment could have been psychological, calming. To this case, Case Kahun 23 is sometimes added, whose heading has not been preserved and whose treatment includes a mouthwash from a fermented decoction of medicinal herbs.

Kahun 33: Toothache *(tiau)*

This case describes another brief, but incompletely preserved, prescription for stopping a toothache that is evidently related to childbirth, perhaps as a consequence of strong clenching of the jawbone. On the day of childbirth, a woman receives a mixture of beans ground with other ingredients, whose names, however, have not been preserved, on her teeth and gums. According to the text, this preparation was tested many times. Violent clenching of the jaw during labor pains can in fact lead to the complication mentioned in this case. The expression *tiau*, used in this case clearly in connection with a cramp of the jaw, apparently disproves Bardinet's theory of tetanus (see above).

Ramesseum IV.A ll. 2–4: Pain of the pubic region and during sexual intercourse

This small fragment of a case is devoted to a woman suffering from pains of the pubic region and pains during sexual intercourse. The physician is to examine the hypogastrium of the woman, but the rest of the text unfortunately cannot be reconstructed.

Ebers 815: Pains

The women's problems described in this case are labeled as pain and suffering, although their cause is not mentioned in the text. A medicinal douche was given with a mixture from milk, the unknown mineral *kesenty,* and acacia leaves, which act as an astringent, hence contract the veins and speed the healing of mucous membranes. The mixture was first left standing overnight and after application was to cool the woman's reproductive system.

Ebers 816: The same

Another remedy for the same problems recommends a mixture from dates, two types of oil, water, and acacia leaves. The treatment method was to be the same.

Ebers 817: Pains of the vulva

This case describes a medicine for pains in the vaginal entry. The mixture for the treatment of the problem was prepared from resin, ochre, incense, acacia leaves, bull's spinal cord, water, the unknown mineral *nehdet*, and the unknown plant *heny-ta*. After mixing all of these ingredients, the blend was used for a douche.

Fever and swellings

Increased body temperature, called fever, is an accompanying symptom of infections or inflammation in various places of the body, hence also in the female reproductive system.

In past times with women who gave birth, bacterial infections often penetrated the female genitals because of unhygienic conditions during or after childbirth. The organism can defend itself against infections by creating a local wall of white blood cells (leukocytes) and antibodies. The course and result of an illness depend on the ratio of the virulence of the microbes to the intensity of the defensive reaction of the organism. If the infection prevails, it can lead to the sepsis of the whole organism, usually ending in death. The origin of the illness called puerperal fever (puerperal sepsis) and the method of how to prevent it by disinfection with chemical means (antisepsis) were discovered in 1847 by the Hungarian obstetrician Ignatius Semmelweis.

Swellings can also occur on various places of the body in pathological processes of entirely different origin: they accompany infections (including puerperal fever), disorders of the venous return in cardiac insufficiency, kidney diseases, and so on.

Kahun 25: Fever

This case deals with a woman who suffers from a fever and whose eyes are bleary. The cause of the illness is not evident. The medication is ground wild carrot mixed with the drink *mesta* and applied for four days, apparently on the woman's private parts. A concurrently recommended treatment is a bath in water that comes from a lake and from another water source, whose specification has not been preserved. The end of the case has unfortunately been destroyed. According to the symptoms, the woman suffering could have been affected by puerperal fever. Ground wild carrot appears also in the cases of postnatal care (Ebers 823) and could positively affect vision, thanks to the content of the orange pigment carotene, from which vitamin A (retinol or axerophthol) is created.

Kahun 15: Swelling of the pubic region

The case deals with a woman with a swollen pubic region. The complete text has not been preserved, and there is also a gap in the place where the diagnosis would be, so the cause of the swelling is not clear. As medicine, the woman is to receive finely ground malachite powder scalded in cow's milk. The end of the case is destroyed, but the number at the end means that the medicine was to be administered for at least three days.

Bleeding and menstruation

Bleeding in women can have a large number of causes, but Egyptian texts in the cases dedicated to bleeding do not mention the causes. It is likely that the majority of the described cases were related to problems connected with menstruation.

Regular female menstrual bleeding or menses (eumenorrhea) is a physiological process of the menstrual cycle, repeating at an interval of usually twenty-eight days. In the ovaries of a woman from puberty until menopause (climacterium), there develop around the maturing eggs covered cavities filled with fluid (ovarian follicles), one of which arches itself above the surface of the ovary. During the thirteenth to fourteenth days of the cycle, the follicle ruptures (ovulation), expels a mature egg, and transforms into a so-called 'yellow body' (corpus luteum). The orifice of the fallopian tube catches this egg with its projections (fimbriae). If fertilization occurs in this (most suitable) period, the corpus luteum changes into a yellow body of pregnancy, producing hormones (corpus luteum graviditatis); if not, it degenerates into scar tissue, and the production of hormones decreases. In the meantime, since the previous menses, the uterine mucous membrane (endometrium) has been prepared by growth, permeation, mucus, and substances for the nourishment of the fertilized egg, which is captured in it. If the egg is not fertilized, the endometrium disintegrates, its surface level separates, and the blood from the torn capillaries results in menstrual bleeding. Blood mixed with fragments of the endometrium and mucus of its glandulae does not coagulate. The entire menstrual cycle is governed hormonally from the pituitary gland.

With menstrual bleeding, its regularity, the amount of blood flow, and duration are usually observed. Fluctuations in these criteria were the subject of medical examination even in antiquity.

Smith *verso* 20: Menstrual problems

This carefully described case deals with delayed menstruation connected with pains of the hypogastrium and an uncertain finding above the navel. According to the diagnosis, it is "stagnation of the blood" *(shenau)* in the womb, but the case does not mention more details or accompanying symptoms, and "stagnation of the blood" (amenorrhea) can be interpreted in various ways. In young girls, it could be a late puberty (primary amenorrhea), mainly caused by developmental faults of the reproductive system; in women over age forty, it could be exhaustion of the embryonic follicles in the ovaries (premature menopause); in a woman of reproductive age, it could be a skipping of menstruation (secondary amenorrhea). The cause could be a beginning pregnancy, neuroendocrine disorders, a condition after a severe illness, or mental stress.

The prescription includes three different medicines, which are to be applied in various ways. The medicine composed of oil, sweet beer, and the unidentified plant *wam* was to be drunk by the patient for four days. At the same time, her womb was to be regularly smeared with a mix of cedar oil, caraway seed, galenite, and myrrh, and if bleeding commenced, oil with the plant "hyena's ear" was applied as well. In addition to that, the woman's private parts were fumigated with myrrh and incense.

Kahun 2: Bleeding from the uterus

This case says that the woman became ill as a consequence of movement of the uterus. The cases of a so-called wandering uterus are a manifestation of the Egyptian opinion of the possible movement of some internal organs in the abdominal cavity. In addition, the affected woman smells like roasted meat and is bleeding from the uterus. This disease was called *nemesu* in Egyptian. Following the homeopathic principle that "similar should be healed with similar" *(similia similibus curantur)*, the treatment lies in the fumigation of the female genitals with something that a woman perceives as the smell of roasted meat, resembling the smell she herself emits. Griffith (1898, 6) interpreted this case as the diagnosis of carcinoma of the uterus (also Nunn 1996, 81), but other authors have doubted his opinion (for example, Grapow 1956, 112). Some specialists (for instance, Westendorf 1992, 194–95) have admitted that it could be cancer of the uterus, while adding that an ancient Egyptian physician could have noticed the typical symptoms of this variety of carcinoma without generally knowing tumors and understanding their malignancy. If that was the case, it was most likely an ulcerating tumor, as is implied by the smell described. It is one of the few pieces of evidence of the knowledge of malignant tumors in ancient Egypt. Their existence is proved by more than fifty paleopathological finds (Strouhal and Němečková 2008, 24–26, 153–54).

Ebers 828: Bleeding

This brief prescription is intended for the "removal" of bleeding. It is relatively difficult to interpret to which disorder the treatment was applied, because the problems of the woman are not specified in any way in the text. Most likely, it was induction of a delayed menstruation. It might have also stopped excessive bleeding by the "removal" of the blood (e.g., Nunn 1996, 197), although heavy menstrual bleeding (menorrhagia) is not directly mentioned in the text. The healing mixture includes onion and wine, which were mixed in equal amounts and applied to the vagina.

Ebers 829: The same

Another prescription for the same problems includes a mixture of equal amounts of acacia leaves, moringa oil, oil, the plant *pakh-seryt*, pea, and honey. It was applied through a douche to the vagina.

Ebers 830: The same

Another preparation for the same problems includes a mixture of fennel and honey, sweet beer, and a greater amount of milk fat. The preparation was to be applied as douches for four days.

Ebers 832: Bleeding

A disorder of bleeding is also connected with pains on one side of the pubic region, which are related to irregularities of menstruation. A bandage with a mixture of onions, muskmelon, and cedar sawdust was to help.

Ebers 833: Stagnation of the blood

This case describes long-lasting amenorrhea, that is, stagnation of the blood, which was believed to happen as a consequence of damaging magic. The healing mixture was prepared from milk and bone marrow, which were boiled and to which juniper berries (an antiseptic, diuretic), Roman cumin (carminative, stimulant), incense, and earth almonds were subsequently added.

Urinary problems

A certain group of cases from the medical texts is devoted to problems connected with urination. Common infections of the urinary tube (urethra) in women (nongonococcal urethritis) can emerge from many causes, for example, by its injury, expulsion of kidney stones (cystolithiasis), and the application of inappropriate douches, but also from eating hot foods or from masturbation, and so on. Besides these common infections, there can also appear a more serious sexual infection of gonorrhea, which in women affects not only the urethra, but also the orifice of the Bartholin's glands in the vaginal opening and cervix, and in a serious ascending form it also affects the endometrium, fallopian tubes, and ovaries. It is an acute infection caused by gonococcal bacteria. It manifests itself with burning or pain during urination, its increased frequency, discharge from the vagina, and cloudy urine. While the occurrence of gonorrhea in ancient Egypt has not yet been proved, it can be assumed, unlike the apparently absent syphilis (Leca 1971, 91).

Kahun 10: Pain during urination

This case describes a disease of the urinary tract that was attributed to a disorder *(khau)* of the womb. As the treatment, it recommends drinking a mixture of 480 ml *(hin)* of beer mulled with pine nuts, beans, and yellow nutsedge for four days. Other than this mixture, the woman was to refrain from eating and drinking for the rest of the day and night. The mixture of medicinal herbs in beer, which has a diuretic effect, could help in purging the urinary tract.

Kahun 34: Pain during urination

Only a small part of this case has been preserved. According to the title, it is pain during urination, most likely as a consequence of an infection of the urinary bladder. The method of treatment has not been preserved. In the conclusion, there is probably advice for preventing further problems for the woman to remain such (healthy?) forever. However, this passage has unfortunately been destroyed.

Ebers 784: Pain during urination

This case describes a preparation that was to be poured into the rectum of a woman. Despite the misleading place of application, however, it was a case of painful urination, and according to the ideas of Egyptian physicians, it led in the body to the transfer of the medicinal substances to the necessary place in the urinary tract. The medicinal mixture included sea salt, sweet beer, honey, and milk fat. Pouring the medicinal mixture into the rectum could also speed the evacuation of a hardened stool and thus perhaps indirectly ease the urination problems.

Ebers 786 + 787: Urination of a clot

This case is intended for women who urinate "something coagulated," probably a blood clot. For the woman, a place on the ground is to be prepared, which is sprinkled with pieces of clay, at night poured over with water, and in the early morning sprinkled with dew. The woman should first sit for a long time on this spot and then for four days over a vessel with oil. It is apparently a case of bleeding in the urinary tract, most likely during an infection of the urinary bladder. The described treatment could have had a purely psychotherapeutic effect.

Ramesseum III.A II. 8: Urination
From this short case, only a part of the title has been preserved, according to which these were instructions for how to correct or induce urination in a woman.

Other women's problems
Besides the above-mentioned issues, women were troubled by a wide range of further problems. In some cases, these could be more serious illnesses of the womb in the form of infections, ulcers, or even cancer. At other times, the causes of the problems were unclear to the doctors and were attributed to the activity of harmful magic. Only a small portion of some cases described in the texts has been preserved; hence it is very difficult to understand their meaning.

Ebers 785: Cooling of the rectum
This preparation is intended for pouring into the rectum. The problems of the patient are not entirely specified; it could have been a painful infection of hemorrhoids. The ingredients included moringa oil, oil, juice from the pulp of carob pods, and honey.

Ebers 812: Discharge
This case treats a discharge from the vagina. A mixture of myrtle and the dregs of excellent beer is applied to the pubic region. The leaves, flowers, and fruits of the myrtle act as an astringent and antiseptic (Manniche 1999, 124), hence the application of myrtle could be effective. The possible causes of the discharge from the vagina include gonorrhea, spread by sexual intercourse, further diseases induced by fungi and yeasts (mycoses), protozoans (for example, trichomoniasis), and various kinds of bacteria, as well as viral diseases (genital herpes or human papillomavirus).

Ebers 813: Infection with ulcers
The preparation described in this case is recommended against "eating away" or "biting" in the womb and for ulcers in the vagina. Nunn interpreted "eating away" as cancer of the womb (1996, 81), but ulcers rather indicate that it

is an ulcerative infection of the vaginal and uterine mucous membranes, which could affect not only a woman both before and after childbirth, but also a non-pregnant woman. The mixture, prepared from fresh dates, cinnamon-tree leaves, and stone from the river bank, was to be pounded and mixed with water, to be left overnight and applied to the vagina.

Ebers 814: The same
Another preparation for the same problems was composed of dates, pig brain, and the *kesenty* mineral. The method of preparation and application was the same.

Ebers 818: *Kemit* and ulcers
The problems described in this case are labeled with the Egyptian expression *kemit*. The reference to ulcers in the vagina could indicate that it is a parallel to Case Ebers 813. The medicinal mixture for the douche was composed of wild carrot, incense, and the mineral *kesenty*.

Ebers 819: The same
Another preparation for the same problems was composed of earth almonds, dates, acacia leaves, and the *kesenty* mineral; water and ass's milk were added as well. The mixture was left to stand overnight and was used for a douche.

Ebers 831: Damage of the womb
This case describes discharge with a blood clot, which is diagnosed as a consequence of "scratching" in the womb. It could be flaking of the endometrium, for example, after a healed infection. The medicine was prepared from Nile clay from a water pump, honey, and galenite, and applied on a cloth tampon.

Ebers 834: Cutting pain in the womb
The preparation recommended in this case was to act on "cutting" in the womb, which might have been an acute infection, manifested through hotness. According to the brief instructions, the treatment was conducted by a douche of a mixture of bull's brain, the *kesenty* mineral, and oil.

Ebers 837: Weakness of the leg
A woman whose legs are weak was to swallow a mixture including sourdough from barley boiled with the unidentified plant *khesau*. The causes of the weakness are not clear, and it could have been a magical preparation.

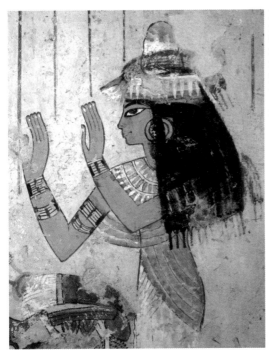

Fig. 42. A woman in a respectful pose is dressed in a fine, pleated gown and ornamented with jewels and lotus flowers, which symbolized resurrection. (Eighteenth Dynasty, tomb of Menna [TT 69] in Sheikh Abd al-Qurna, photo: M. Zemina)

Ebers 169: Evil magic

This case is part of the group of cases in the Ebers Papyrus that are to prevent harmful magic. The medicinal mixture, which was composed of date pulp, oil, and yeast and was to be drunk, could influence an unspecified illness of some abdominal organ. Although the problems from which the woman suffered are not described in the text, the expression "her belly refuses" could imply intestinal problems or perhaps infertility.

Ebers 174: Evil magic

Another prescription for unclear problems included a number of ingredients like coriander, the plant *ibu*, sorghum, fruits of the *shasha*, and pellitory. These ingredients were to be boiled with honey and given to the woman to eat before sleeping.

Kahun 14: Fragment of a case

A thirsty woman should be given an infused and fermented herbal decoction. It is only a fragment of the prescription; we thus do not know its full wording, the causes of the problems, or the full composition of the medicine.

Kahun 18: Fragment of a case

This is a fragment of the prescription for the unknown disease *sehau*, for which no description of the woman's symptoms has been preserved. A medicinal preparation composed of milk and other ingredients that have not been preserved was used for wiping the woman's private parts.

Ramesseum IV.C II. 1–2: Fragment of a case

Only a small part of the last sentence of this case has been preserved. Hence, it is not clear what problems afflicted the woman who was treated. According to the preserved part of the text, a medicine in the form of tartlets was to be prepared.

Support of conception

From time immemorial, people have known the role of male semen, and the Egyptians expressed themselves on conception simply: "He slept with his wife and she became pregnant." We also find detailed descriptions of sexual acts in the legends recounting the divine origin of several rulers. They were usually written down for political reasons, to strengthen the claim of the relevant pharaoh to the Egyptian throne, and described how the supreme god Amun transformed into the form of the king-father, visited the queen-mother, and conceived the future king with her (fig. 43). The child thus was the son of a god and also of the king.

One of the significant Egyptian gods was the god of fertility Min, from whose divine erect sexual organ semen sprayed (fig. 44) (Wilkinson 2003, 115–16). According to Egyptian ideas, semen originated in the bones and two tubes brought it to each of the testicles.

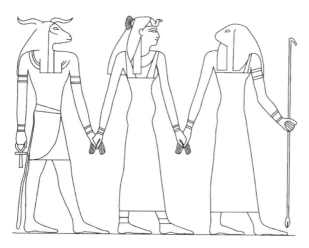

Fig. 43. The god Khnum and goddess Heqet lead the mother of Queen Hatshepsut to childbirth. Queen Ahmose conceived after she was visited by the god Amun, who took on the form of her royal husband Thutmose I. (Eighteenth Dynasty, Hatshepsut's temple at Deir al-Bahari, drawing: H. Vymazalová after Naville 1896, pl. XLIX)

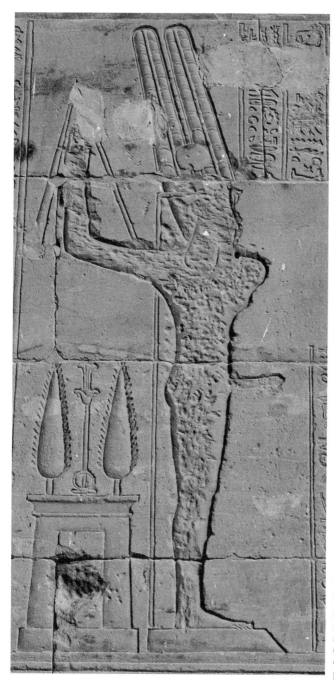

Fig. 44. The god Min, with
an erect phallus, was the
god of fertile strength;
behind him, we can see his
symbolic plant, lettuce, considered to be an aphrodisiac
and signifying male fertility.
(Ptolemaic Period, temple
on the Island of Philae,
photo: M. Megahed)

The Egyptians did not know the precise anatomy of female internal sexual organs, and they perhaps derived a lot from observation of the relevant parts of female animals during disembowelment after slaughter. They thus noticed that the fallopian tubes are open to the abdominal cavity. Since according to Egyptian ideas the digestive tract, beginning at the mouth, also opened in this way, the Egyptians came to the opinion that both anatomical systems were hence connected. They thus also saw the possibility of conception through practicing non-classical methods of sexual intercourse. This idea was already reflected in the ancient myth of the creation of the world by the creator god Atum, who first conceived his children—the god Shu and goddess Tefnut—by swallowing his own semen. Ideas of a similar character could also have been invoked by rare cases of extrauterine pregnancy, when the fetus gets a foothold elsewhere than in the uterus.

Kahun 20: Conception

The text of this case has been only partially preserved and is very unclear. According to the title, it deals with a woman who has used a preparation for conception, but the precise description of the problems has not been preserved. It could be care after a spontaneous miscarriage, when regular menstruation should return (see also Westendorf 1999, 426). A prescription is attached for a strained, fermented decoction from medicinal herbs and milk fat. Fumigation with a mixture of incense, oil, dates, and sweet beer is further recommended. The conclusion of the case mentions a preparation intended for oral hygiene, which might have been added to the medicinal mixture as well.

Carlsberg VIII, 1: Achieving conception

Only a very small part of this case has been preserved. Quite clearly, it is a prescription for achieving conception, but unfortunately neither its ingredients nor the method of application has been preserved.

Prevention of conception

Although Egyptians loved children, and their own offspring were one of life's priorities for them, not every pregnancy was wanted. Sometimes a woman did not want to become pregnant, either because she had already borne several children or because pregnancy was undesirable for other reasons, for example with prostitutes. From experience, women knew that as long as they were breastfeeding, the likelihood of conception was reduced. Perhaps for that reason it was a habit to breastfeed for as long as three years in Egypt (Strouhal 1992, 23). Besides this unreliable method, however, the preserved medicinal texts describe a wide range of preparations against conception, which utilized various ingredients of herbal, animal, and mineral origin. Some preparations were applied in herbal tampons and placed directly in the vagina; others were smeared on the whole vulva.

The effectiveness of these preparations is questionable. Of the ingredients that are mentioned in the preserved cases, a certain effect could have been achieved by honey, which acts as a spermicide. The effects of other herbal ingredients are hard to judge, because some of them have not yet been identified.

It is interesting that none of the preparations in the preserved texts was administered orally, which could indicate that despite the imprecise ideas of the anatomical arrangement of the sexual organs, Egyptian women proceeded from empirically verified methods in the use of contraception. In other areas, for instance the testing of fertility (see below), much more superstition is apparent.

Kahun 21: Preventing conception

This case describes a preparation that was to prevent conception. Although the text has not been preserved in its entirety, its parallel can be found in the following case, Ramesseum IV.C ll. 2–3. For preventing conception, this case recommends an herbal decoction mixed with crocodile dung. This disgusting ingredient could have worked magically. According to some opinions, however, crocodile dung also could have had a spermicidal effect (Robins 1993, 80), and after grinding in a liquid it formed a mushroom-like structure (Watterson 1991, 88) that could capture the moving sperm on its surface.

Ramesseum IV.C ll. 2–3: Preventing conception

This preparation, which was to prevent a woman from becoming pregnant, is similar to the means from the prescription in the previous case, Kahun 21. The text has been preserved only partially, but it is clear from it that the ingredient is crocodile dung, which was probably mixed with something liquid (a decoction of medicinal plants) and was used to saturate a tampon of plant fibers. A tampon inserted at the orifice of the uterus (in the vaginal part of the cervix) could act as a pessary, a not-very-reliable obstacle to the movement of sperm.

Kahun 22: Preventing conception

Another preparation for the same purpose presents 480 ml *(hin)* of honey and natron mash as the contraceptive means. It is not entirely clear whether the two ingredients were mixed, or whether the private parts were smeared only with honey and a woman did so seated above a vessel containing a mash from natron. Honey has proven spermicidal effects and could in reality act against conception; natron could osmotically help create a hostile environment for sperm in the womb and in the vagina.

Kahun 23: Preventing conception (?)

The description of another means for the same purpose has been preserved only partially. The mixture includes a fermented decoction of medicinal herbs, probably with some other ingredient, which is unknown today. It was applied to the woman's private parts. Some experts connect this case with Case Kahun 24 (see p. 145) and consider both as parts of one case.

Ebers 783: Preventing conception

This prescription presents a preparation that can prevent a woman from becoming pregnant in the long term. The text mentions that the effectiveness may last for one, two, or three years, which most likely means that the preparation could be used without limitations. The mixture includes some part *(kaa)* of the acacia plant, the pulp of carob pods, and dates, which were ground and mixed with 480 ml *(hin)* of honey. The preparation was applied directly into the vagina using a tampon of plant fibers. The spermicidal effects of honey could be enhanced further by the plant components mentioned.

Berlin 192: Preventing conception (?)

This case has not been preserved in its entirety, but it seems that it was a preparation to help prevent conception in a woman. The woman's private parts were to be fumigated with sorghum, and moreover a mixture of equal parts of oil, celery, and sweet beer was to be prepared for her. The woman was to drink the boiled mixture for four mornings for her to "release it."

Tests of fertility and pregnancy

Bearing children was an unwritten obligation for Egyptian women. It is therefore no surprise that we also find in medical papyri tests revealing a woman's ability to be impregnated and give birth. These instructions are numerous in the texts and describe various methods for determining whether a woman is fertile, or even already pregnant. They are usually introduced by a more or less brief variation of the phrase "how to recognize a woman who will give birth and a woman who will not give birth." This question was naturally very important for Egyptian society, because the inability of a woman to produce children was a greatly feared malady, which could even lead to divorce. Egyptian women were therefore very afraid of sterility, and their desire to become pregnant was captured by statues of pregnant women as early as the Predynastic Period.

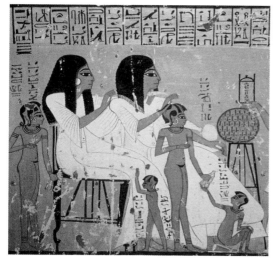

Fig. 45. An image of a loving family, with an older married couple surrounded by their four grandchildren. The three girls and small boy are depicted nude and with the so-called sidelock of youth. (Twentieth Dynasty, tomb of Inerkhau at Deir al-Medina [TT 359], photo: M. Zemina)

Egyptians loved children very much, and begetting children and preserving the family was one of their essential priorities (fig. 45). *The Maxims of Ani* (Eighteenth Dynasty) says: "Take a wife while you are young so that she may make a son for you. She should bear for you while you are youthful, it is proper to make people" (Lichtheim 1976, 136). The importance of the fertility of women is also emphasized by the evidence of small domestic shrines for the veneration of the gods of fertility, such as Taweret, Hathor, or the dwarf god Bes (fig. 46). Examples are known from archaeological excavations in the village of Deir al-Medina from the New Kingdom and also in Akhetaten (today's Tell al-Amarna), the residential city of the reformer king Akhenaten from the second half of the Eighteenth Dynasty. Although some cases of adoption have also been documented (Robins 1993, 77–78), to have one's own child was yearningly anticipated in the ancient world.

The determination of the fertility of a woman by the methods described in the papyri Kahun, Berlin, and Carlsberg VIII is very interesting. According to their headings, these methods were to reveal whether a woman will give birth or will never give birth. Some of the methods are based on the administration of a certain medication orally or through the vagina; others proceed from a judgment of the color of the eyes, while still others are based on pouring the urine of the examined woman on grains. The effectiveness of the methods is largely questionable, and some of them reflect the idea that the cause of infertility could be a disruption of the communication between the digestive tract and the reproductive system.

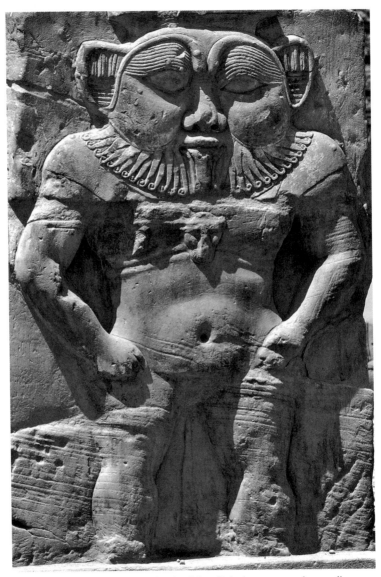

Fig. 46. The god Bes, with a lion's head and dwarf's body, was a popular guardian of young children and patron of happy family life. (Ptolemaic Period, Birth House in the temple of Hathor at Dendara, photo: M. Megahed)

In some cases, the tests evaluating the ability of a woman to conceive and bear a child could reveal an already ongoing pregnancy, and could thus also be used as tests of the state of the pregnancy. That is probably the case with the method of measuring the pulse or examination of the breasts and color of the skin, which sometimes can reveal pregnancy in a woman. Some tests even deal with determining the sex of the unborn child.

Kahun 26: Test of fertility

This case describes a method of how to distinguish a fertile woman from an infertile one. The woman is to be given a mixture of oil and other ingredients, which have not been preserved in the text. This is followed by an examination of her breasts; if their *metu* are enlarged, the woman will give birth. The word *metu* in Egyptian medicine meant blood vessels, nerves, and other oblong tubular and tube-like shapes between which Egyptian physicians did not precisely distinguish. In this case, it could have been the swollen mammary glands or expanded blood vessels (veins) of a woman who is already pregnant. If the breasts appear to the physician as unhealthy (?), the woman should be able to conceive later. Another possibility is that the blood vessels will be colored, but the text has been damaged at the conclusion, and hence the prognosis for this possibility has not been preserved. A similar method is described in Case Berlin 196.

Berlin 196: Test of fertility

According to this case, the woman's breasts, arms, and shoulders are to be smeared with fresh oil before she goes to bed. Early the next morning, it is necessary to examine carefully the *metu* (blood vessels) on her body. If they seem uncompressed, literally 'unsunken,' hence if they are easily visible and filled with blood, the woman will be able to conceive children. If her blood vessels are hard to see (literally 'sunken') and are not distinguishable from the surrounding body, something is not right with the woman. If the blood vessels are green and dark, the woman will be able to conceive later. The instructions are similar to the previous case, Kahun 26.

Kahun 27: Test of fertility

Another method for determining a woman's ability to conceive has also not been preserved in its entirety. The woman was to be seated on the ground, which had been sprinkled with dregs of sweet beer, and eat fruit. The text is, however, damaged and we do not know the precise wording. If the woman began to vomit, it meant that she would have children or was already pregnant.

Moreover, the number of children was to correspond to the number of vomitings, but if the woman did not begin vomiting, she was considered infertile.

Kahun 28: Test of fertility

Another method includes the use of onions. The text has been preserved only partially, and it seems that it was a variant of Case Carlsberg VIII, 4, where the onion was placed in the woman's vagina, after which it was established whether a stench came from the breath (nose) of the woman or not (see below).

Carlsberg VIII, 4: Test of fertility

This case is similar to Case Kahun 28, when an onion was placed in the vagina and the next day it was determined whether the woman emitted an odor from her mouth. If she did not, she was considered infertile. This case refers to the ancient Egyptian belief that the reproductive system was connected with the digestive tract. The stench of the onion thus proved the patency of the routes that were considered necessary for the production of a child.

Kahun 29: Test of fertility

Another method recognizes a woman's ability to conceive by the fact that she feels pain if the physician pulls her by a lip while his other hand holds her by the shoulder. According to the earlier Griffith translation, the physician is to strike the woman on the mouth, but the verb *nedjer* means rather 'to grasp, to seize.' If the woman does not feel pain, she is considered infertile. The Egyptian expression for 'a lip' can, however, mean also the labia in the vulva, which in this case might be more fitting.

Kahun 30: Test of fertility

This very damaged text for determining a fertile woman is introduced by a magical incantation, which was apparently to enhance the effect of the method applied. The incantation refers to the god Horus and the calf of Horus, but its wording is not entirely clear, because it is interrupted by many tears in the papyrus. A woman is considered fertile if something (the text has not been preserved) comes out of her nose or her private parts. The conditions describing her infertility have unfortunately not been preserved.

Kahun 31: Test of fertility

Another method for determining a fertile woman has been preserved only from a small part. It apparently lies in a visual examination of the female's face. If something in her eyes does not seem right to the physician, the woman is infertile. If the woman's face looks healthy (Griffith 1898, 10 translates it as 'green') but there is something strange about it, she is able to bear a son, but the text is incomplete here, and the sense of the case is not entirely clear.

Kahun 32: Fragment of a case
This text is a fragment. As with Case Kahun 29 (see above), the physician is to place a fingertip on the woman's shoulder and observe her reaction.

Berlin 193: Test of fertility
According to this method for determining a fertile woman, a mixture of watermelon with human breast milk was prepared for drinking. If the woman then vomited, she could have children. If flatulence resulted, she was considered infertile. The breast milk comprising a part of the preparation was to come from a woman who was the mother of a male child. This detail probably reflected the fact that in ancient Egyptian society, as in many others, parents desired mainly boys.

Berlin 194: Test of fertility
Another method utilizes the same preparation; in this case, however, it is not given to the woman to drink but is applied as a douche of her private parts. A fertile woman vomits; an infertile woman is revealed by flatulence.

Berlin 195: Test of fertility
This case describes another method for determining the fertility of a woman who has not yet given birth. Her private parts are to be fumigated with hippopotamus dung. If the woman urinates and defecates or feels flatulence, she is considered fertile. If she feels nothing, she cannot have children.

Carlsberg VIII, 5: Test of fertility
This case for determining a fertile woman utilizes—just like Case Berlin 195—fumigation of the woman's private parts. The text has not been preserved in its entirety, so it is not clear which substance was to be used for fumigation this time. A woman is considered fertile if she vomits and infertile if she experiences flatulence.

Berlin 197: Test of fertility or pregnancy
This case determines whether a woman can have a child by checking the pulse. The woman's arm is exercised and then palpated from all sides to determine whether the arteries *(metu)* pulse properly. If so, she will become pregnant.

Berlin 198: Test of fertility

In this case, the woman's fertility is determined from the color of her eyes. During the examination, the woman is to stand in the doorway so that enough light falls on her. A woman who can have children should have both eyes of the same color. If each of her eyes has a different color, namely "like Asians" (blue or otherwise light) and "like Nubians" (dark), then she is considered infertile. The same method is also recorded in Case 6 on the Carlsberg VIII Papyrus (see below).

Carlsberg VIII, 6: Test of fertility

This case describes the same method as Case Berlin 198. A woman is considered fertile if both of her eyes have the same color.

Berlin 199: Test of fertility, pregnancy, and determination of the child's sex

This case describes another method of determining fertility and establishing the sex of an unborn child. Each day, the woman is to pour her urine on barley and wheat (and also dates and plain sand). If the plants sprout and grow, the woman can have children. If the plants do not grow, the woman is considered infertile. Pouring the urine on the dates and sand could have been a verification of the test.

Egyptians connected sprouting grains, the manifestation of new life, with the formation of a child in a woman's womb. This test could actually reveal an already ongoing pregnancy, as been experimentally verified, with an accuracy of twenty-eight out of forty samples (Ghalioungui, Khalil, and Ammar 1963). Today, we know that the urine of pregnant women contains the hormone human chorionic gonadotropin, whose presence can be tested immunologically (Kobilková et al. 2005, 217).

The same test was allegedly also able to determine the sex of the unborn child. Barley was connected with the birth of a boy, because its name in Egyptian was of masculine gender, whereas a girl was connected with wheat, labeled with an expression of feminine gender (Watterson 1991, 87). Modern experiments have not proved the efficacy of this aspect of the test, however. The same method is also described in Case 3 on Papyrus Carlsberg VIII.

Carlsberg VIII, 3: Test of fertility, pregnancy, and determination of the child's sex

This case is similar to Case Berlin 199. Every day, the woman is to pour her urine on barley and wheat in a cloth bag. Various results of the experiment correspond to various possibilities of pregnancy. If both crops grow at once, it means that she will give birth many times; if only barley grows, she will have a boy; if only wheat grows, she will have a girl; and if they do not grow at all, she apparently is not pregnant.

Carlsberg VIII, 2: Test of fertility and prognosis of survival
Unfortunately, only a very small part of this case has been preserved. It speaks of sand from the coastline and fabric bags, which apparently were to be filled with dates and onto which the woman was to pour her urine (?). The prognosis is based on whether worms appear in the bags. This method determined whether the woman was fertile (or pregnant), but also whether the child would be viable.

Carlsberg VIII, 7: Test of fertility
According to these instructions, the woman whose ability to have children is being determined is to be given a mixture of dates, mashed dates, and wine to drink. The text has unfortunately not been preserved in its entirety. If the woman feels bad, she cannot have children; in the opposite case, she can conceive.

Kahun 19: Prenatal prognosis
Unfortunately, only a very small part of this case has been preserved. According to the title, it is probably a pregnancy test based on the appearance or absence of a menstrual period, or a determination of the date of the childbirth.

Pregnancy
During pregnancy, the Egyptians took care that a woman ate enough food of good quality and thus ensured her child's health and beauty. As with the women of today's fellaheen (Egyptian agricultural workers), a pregnant woman was to avoid looking at unpleasant things and, on the contrary, was to endeavor to come into contact with positive and beautiful phenomena (Watterson 1991, 87).

A normal pregnancy, lasting on average 269 days from fertilization (or 282 days from the first day of the last menstruation), takes place without complications for a healthy and mentally balanced woman. Pregnancy is a physiological process governed by hormones and the nerve centers that protect the woman and the developing fetus from disorders. However, a whole range of the latter can appear in its course. One of the serious complications mentioned in the papyri is bleeding, which is a sign of a threat to the pregnancy by miscarriage or premature childbirth (fig. 47).

Attempts at preventing premature childbirth were based on magical acts. The causes of bleeding, which Egyptian healers did not precisely understand,

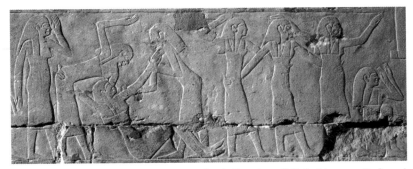

Fig. 47. Pregnant women do not appear very often in Egyptian reliefs. In this scene of a funeral procession, some of them faint under the strain of the emotional experience. (Sixth Dynasty, tomb of Ankhmahor at Saqqara, photo: M. Zemina)

were attributed to the influence of unknown, inauspicious powers or even the harmful activity of dead persons, who according to Egyptian ideas could intervene in the life of the living in both a positive and a negative way. The solution was closing the birth canal with a knot of plant fibers, referring to the magical knot of Isis, *tyet* (fig. 48), which symbolized the tampon that the god Atum tied in Isis's womb to protect her developing son Horus from the devastating intervention of the hostile god Seth. The *tyet* was therefore used as a popular protective amulet in relation to birth or rebirth after death and was

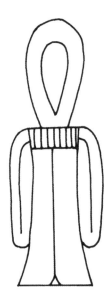

usually produced from carnelian or jasper. The invocation of various deities over the pregnant woman during the preparation of this tampon was to ensure its magical effectiveness. The gods mentioned in the magical incantations refer to the myth of the birth of the god Horus, who was born to the goddess Isis in the papyrus bushes of the Nile Delta. With the assistance of other gods, namely her sister Nephthys or Anubis, Isis hid him and protected him from the god Seth.

Fig. 48. The knot of Isis, *tyet*, was often produced as a protective amulet from carnelian or jasper, which have the color of blood. It is discussed in spell 156 of the *Book of the Dead*. (Drawing: J. Malátková)

London 40: Preventing bleeding

The beginning of this prescription has not been preserved, but it seems that along with two other cases it is an incantation for stopping bleeding in a woman. It is very likely bleeding during pregnancy, and the treatment is based on magical methods. The incantation mentioning the gods from Heliopolis was to be delivered above a linen tampon with four knots, which was smeared with pork liver and placed in the woman's rectum. The magical effect of the incantation was enhanced by special ingredients (a swallow's feathers, ass hair, turtle liver). This method refers to the idea that the digestive tract, accessible through the anus, was connected in the belly with the reproductive system of a woman. The conclusion of the text says that this magical method should also "strengthen the egg," in other words, fix the fetus in the mother's uterus.

London 41: Preventing bleeding

Another preparation against bleeding in pregnancy again utilizes a linen tampon with one knot, which was, however, in this case placed in the woman's vagina. The magical incantation describes how the god Anubis stopped a flood on the territory of the goddess Tayet. The goddess Tayet was the patron goddess of fabrics and hence could increase the magical power of the linen tampon. For her protective abilities, she was sometimes identified with the goddess Isis or Hathor (Wilkinson 2003, 168; Janák 2005, 172–73). The jackal god Anubis protected Isis and the child Horus when they were hiding in the papyrus bushes of the Nile Delta (Wilkinson 2003, 187–90). Analogously to the Nile flood, Anubis could magically stop the flood of blood from the genitals of the pregnant woman and thus ensure the effect of the tampon and protect "what is in her," that is, the fetus.

London 42: Preventing bleeding

This case is intended for the same purpose. The bleeding is explicitly attributed to the magic by which some dead person or demon tried to hurt the woman. The protective magical incantation again mentions the goddess Tayet and calls on the god Anubis to provide protection and expel "what is in her," that is, the bad magic. The linen tampon with two knots was placed in the vagina.

London 45: Preventing bleeding

In this case, the magical incantation is to cause the vagina to close and thus stop bleeding. It refers to Sekhathor, the celestial cow identified with Isis and Hathor, who fed with her milk the Egyptian ruler as well as all of the people. She was identified with Isis and Hathor (Janák 2005, 153), and in this incantation thus fulfilled a protective function.

Childbirth

Egyptian women gave birth often, normally every two to three years; in between, the three years of breastfeeding more or less hormonally protected them from a new pregnancy. Childbirth could take place at home or in a specially prepared shelter in the garden or on the roof of the house, so that the mother in childbed would be separated from the normal domestic hustle and bustle. We know of depictions of such structures from the New Kingdom, and it is possible that after childbirth a woman went through a special purification before she returned to her community (Robins 1993, 84).

According to ancient Egyptian belief, the mother was identified with the goddess Isis, mother of the god Horus, which was to provide magical protection for her and the newborn child. Women gave birth on their knees, as is usually the case with today's Egyptian villagers, or seated on a pad of two bricks separated by a gap. A birth brick has recently been discovered for the first time by the American Pennsylvania–Yale–Institute of Fine Arts expedition during their exploration of a palace from the end of the Thirteenth Dynasty in south Abydos (Wegner 2002 and 2009). It was decorated on all sides by magical images, which were to ensure the protection of the expectant mother and the child (fig. 49). There were also 'labor chairs' *(meskhenet)*, first of unfired bricks, later also of wood (Watterson 1991, 90). The child being delivered is usually depicted with the head and the upper limbs emerging first, as is confirmed by the hieroglyphic symbols for childbirth, and this position corresponds to the advanced phase of normal childbirth (fig. 50).

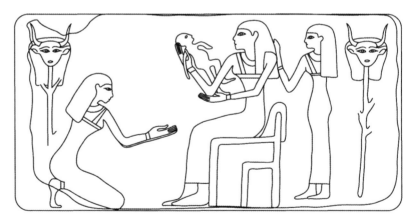

Fig. 49. A birth brick with a depiction of a mother with child after a successful birth. The image was to protect the mother and newborn child from evil. (Thirteenth Dynasty, Abydos, drawing: H. Vymazalová after Wegner 2002, 2009)

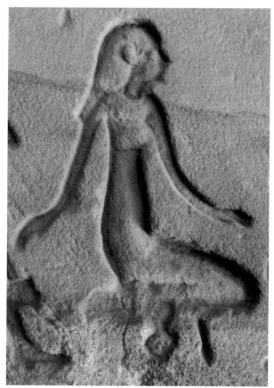

Fig. 50. Hieroglyphic sign representing a woman giving birth. The small head and upper limbs of the child are already emerging from the womb. (Ptolemaic Period, inscription from the temple of Esna, photo: M. Megahed)

During childbirth, the woman was probably assisted by older and more experienced women from her milieu or by midwives, whose profession, however, has not been reliably attested in Egypt. The reliefs on royal monuments (fig. 51) and written evidence describing the birth of kings capture goddesses in the role of birth assistants, particularly Isis and her sister Nephthys, next to them also Heqet with a frog's head and Meskhenet. Magical protection could additionally be assured for the mother in childbed by the goddesses Hathor or Neith, who are often identified with Isis for their protective abilities. Hathor was, moreover, the goddess of fertility and sexuality, and women often invoked her when they had labor pains (Robins 1993, 82–83).

A popular patroness of pregnant, delivering, and breastfeeding women was the goddess Taweret, depicted in the form of a pregnant hippopotamus (fig. 52). Sometimes she is holding in her front hooves a magical knife or Isis's magical knot, *tyet*. The expectant mother could receive additional help from the god of knowledge and wisdom, Thoth, depicted as an ibis or baboon. Labor pains were lessened by the breath of the god Amun, who came in the form of

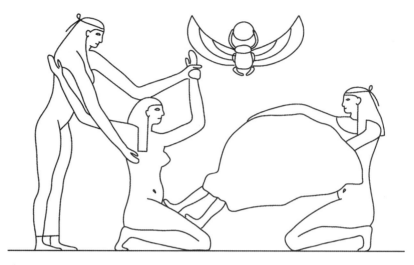

Fig. 51. A depiction of the birth of Queen Cleopatra, rendered by artists from Napoleon's expedition to Egypt. The figure of the child is almost entirely destroyed; the queen is assisted by midwife goddesses. (Ptolemaic Period, temple of Armant, drawing: H. Vymazalová after Néret 2001, p. 67)

a cooling northern breeze. On the abdomen of the birthing woman, the assistants sometimes placed a 'magical knife' of ivory carved into a semicircle and covered with engraving of the protective gods, but also harmful snakes, lions, crocodiles, fantastic animals, and demons. The protective gods included also the chondrodystrophic dwarf god Bes, who protected not only mothers in childbirth but also their family and household (see fig. 46).

The umbilical cord was not cut until the child had been cleaned and washed and after the birth of the placenta. There is no evidence of ligation of the umbilical cord, so they apparently waited for a natural stoppage of the blood's circulation. The placenta and umbilical cord also played an important role in mythology. According to the *Book of the Dead* (Spell No. 17), cutting of the umbilical cord had religious significance and meant a freeing from evil and wicked things (Goelet 1994, 34). The placenta and the umbilical cord were considered as the residence of an alter ego or double of the child. Egyptian villagers to this day call the placenta *al-walad al-tani* ('the second child'). They sometimes preserved the placenta in a dried state for an entire lifetime, and it occasionally even followed them to the grave. A woman could ensure the continuation of her fertility by hiding the placenta under the threshold of the house and then crossing over it repeatedly (three, five, or seven times) (Watterson 1991, 92). Today's countrywomen in Upper Egypt believe that the

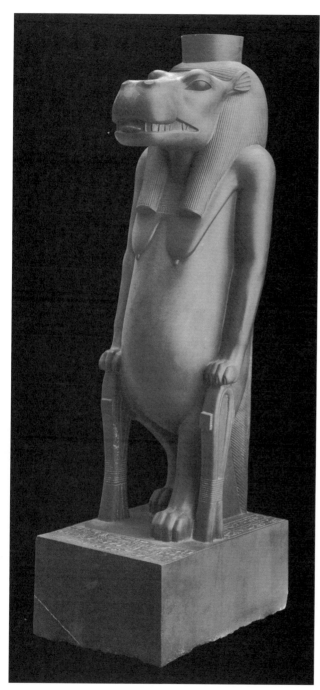

Fig. 52. The goddess Taweret, in the form of a female hippopotamus, was a popular protector of women in pregnancy and childbirth. The ancient Egyptians observed that hippopotamus mothers cared for their offspring carefully, teaching them to swim and protecting them. (Twenty-sixth Dynasty, Egyptian Museum, Cairo [CG 39194], photo: S. Vannini)

placenta must be thrown in the waters of the Nile, and whoever throws it is to smile so that the child will be constantly happy. It is recommended that a woman who cannot conceive place a fresh placenta on her genitals, which will help her become pregnant. This superstition, most likely reflecting the ancient Egyptian belief in the magical power of the placenta, has been maintained in the Egyptian rural milieu to this day.

Physicians did not attend normal childbirths, and gynecology and obstetrics are missing among their specializations. Apparently, a physician was called for childbirth only in exceptional and complicated cases. Birth assistants may have asked for the advice of a physician when it was necessary to accelerate a long-running (protracted) childbirth and hence save the child and mother. Besides childbirth with a normal course *(hetep)*, complicated childbirth *(bened)* and protracted childbirth *(wedef)* are also described in the texts.

In every childbirth, a woman risked death from puerperal fever as a consequence of the unhygienic environment, washing of the female genitalia with polluted water, or the unclean hands of the birth assistants. Heavy bleeding from the female genitalia could cause exsanguination; the fetus could become stuck in the birth canal; if the woman's pelvis was too narrow or the uterus feeble, it could lead to retention of the placenta, pregnancy seizures or convulsions (eclampsia), and other pathological processes. The traces of difficult childbirths and labor complications can be found on the skeletal remains of women, and the remains of numerous newborns from many Egyptian graves confirm how risky childbirth was in ancient times without modern medical care. The dangers of childbirth were reflected in the short average life of adult women as compared to men, whereas the situation is the opposite today in developed countries with modern obstetric care. As a rule, ancient Egyptian women died several years earlier than men. At the same time, not all newborn children survived the danger of childbirths complicated by mechanical problems, or even more frequently by infections. Every third to fourth child did not even live to its first birthday.

While we do not encounter evidence of severe complications in childbirth in the texts, the preserved skeletal remains are often very eloquent. Princess Hehenhet, buried in the funerary complex of Pharaoh Nebhepetre Mentuhotep II (Eleventh Dynasty) in Deir al-Bahari, had a very narrow pelvis, and during a hard childbirth a tear appeared between the vagina and the bladder (vesico-vaginal fistula) (Majno 1975, 115–16). A difficult childbirth could also be caused by a prolapse of the womb externally. Repeated difficult childbirths marked the pelvis of Queen Mutnedjmet, wife of King Horemheb of the Eighteenth

Dynasty, whose skeletal remains were discovered in his tomb in Saqqara. What was probably fatal for the queen was childbirth at an age of forty to forty-five years, in the attempt to ensure an heir to the throne for the land, and among her bones, dispersed by thieves, there lay also the small bones of the mature fetus (Strouhal 2008, 1–4).

When the divine birth assistants from the above-mentioned Westcar Papyrus (Erman 1890) found Lady Rudjdjedet in labor pains, they told her husband: "Let [us] see her, for we are knowledgeable about childbirth" (Simpson 2003, 22). The goddesses hence knew methods (and means) that could ease and accelerate childbirth, and such instructions are recorded also in the preserved texts. The relevant prescriptions include a great number of herbal ingredients and minerals, which were to have a positive effect on the course of childbirth, but the significance of the majority of them is unfortunately not known to us, and thus it is not possible to evaluate their real medical efficacy. In addition to other ingredients, they used strong beer and wine, which thanks to the alcohol content could lower the pain threshold.

It is possible that the preparations in some cases within this group, particularly with the instructions in the Ebers Papyrus, could be used for the premature termination of a pregnancy (Nunn 1996, 194). Such means were certainly in demand even in ancient times, because unwanted pregnancies have occurred from time immemorial. Nevertheless, the texts do not express themselves entirely clearly, and we do not know many of the ingredients that are mentioned, so abortions conducted by Egyptian abortion doctors cannot be proved (or disproved).

Book for Mother and Child G: Protection during childbirth
This magical incantation was to help a woman to bear a child without anything bad happening. It refers to a sacred place, the divine water canal and royal lake with which the child is magically connected.

Ramesseum IV.C ll. 17–24: Protection of the expectant mother
The introductory part of this case describes a method for judging the viability of a newborn, which is verified on the day the child is born (see pp. 188–91). An incantation follows that is to magically ensure the protection of the mother during childbirth. The incantation is aimed particularly against the activity of a dead person (or a demon) with sexual intentions, but the wording of this incantation has not been preserved entirely, which means that it is hard to comprehend. Besides other things, the incantation says that no wrongs should happen to the mother in labor.

Ramesseum IV.C ll. 28–30: Easing childbirth

This case contains a magical incantation that was to help a woman during childbirth. It refers to the goddess Nephthys, sister of Isis, and to the Great, which may refer to the mother goddess in the form of a cow. Along with the incantation, the expectant mother was to be aided by an ointment applied on the crown of the head, but the composition of the ointment was not a part of the text.

Ebers 797: Starting childbirth

This prescription was applied for a woman "to give on the ground" and probably was to ease the beginning of childbirth after the labor pains began. This was to be aided by the *niaia* plant, upon which the expectant mother was to be seated. It is less likely that these are instructions to induce an abortion (Nunn 1996, 194). The understanding of this case would certainly be assisted if it were possible to translate the name of the *niaia* plant, which was given to the woman to relax or to release the fetus from the womb.

Ebers 798: Easing childbirth

This prescription "for everything that is in a woman's belly to come out" was apparently to ease childbirth. The recommended mixture was prepared from mashed sherds of the vessel *hin*, which were mixed with oil and poured into the vagina. This mixture could be intended instead as a preparation for inducing childbirth or cleaning the womb of the remnants of the placenta, but the drastic-looking method could also imply inducing an abortion.

Ebers 799: The same

Another prescription for easing childbirth includes dates, salt, and oil. Heating the mixture to body temperature provided a more pleasant feeling when taking the medicine, which was to be drunk entirely.

Ebers 800: Easing childbirth

This prescription was to ensure that the child was released more easily from the uterus. The prescription included equal amounts of sea salt, white wheat, and the female rush plant, and the mixture was applied to the hypogastrium of the mother in labor.

Ebers 801: The same

Another prescription to ease childbirth was composed of equal amounts of trigonella and honey, and the mixture was to be drunk for one day. Trigonella stimulates lactation, helps heal inflammation, and contains many vitamins. Combined with honey, it thus could have a very positive effect on the mother in labor.

Ebers 802: The same
The prescription made for the mother in labor in this text is composed of equal amounts of fennel, incense, resin, strong beer, fresh trigonella, and fly droppings. The ingredients were to be mixed and applied in the form of a suppository in the vagina. The strong beer could relieve the pain of the mother in labor; the trigonella supported lactation and healing.

Ebers 803: The same
Another prescription for the same included the equal amounts of incense and oil; this mixture was to be used to massage the woman's belly.

Ebers 804: The same
Childbirth could be eased also by a mixture of equal amounts of the *niaia* plant, the unknown mineral *kesenty*, and wine, which was to be used for four days. The first of these ingredients is known already from Case Ebers 797 (see above). What is surprising is the relatively long period of the application of the preparation. If it was a preparation to ease childbirth, the labor pains probably lasted quite long, and the mother must have already been very exhausted. Yet it is also possible that the preparation was to induce an abortion. The pains were to be lessened by the use of wine.

Ebers 805: The same
Another prescription for the mother in labor included equal amounts of the fruits of the *ished* tree and strong beer. The preparation was to be applied to the woman's private parts. Strong beer as one of the ingredients (see Ebers 802 above) was to lower the pain threshold.

Ebers 806: The same
Another prescription for easing childbirth recommended equal amounts of juniper berries, the *niaia* plant, and cedar resin. The mixture was worked into the form of a suppository and applied in the vagina.

Ebers 807: The same
For a mother in labor, it was also possible to prepare a mixture of equal amounts of cedar oil, strong beer, and oil, to which a certain part *(nis)* of a

turtle and beetles were added. The ingredients were to be mashed and applied to the mother. The beer had an effect on the pain, the cedar oil worked as an antiseptic, and the turtle and beetle ingredients were most likely of a magical nature.

Book for Mother and Child F: Easing childbirth

This magical incantation was to help unfasten the child from the body of its mother in order to ease childbirth. It calls on the goddess Meskhenet, who helped expectant mothers during childbirth and cared for newborns. The child received a soul and spirit from the god of the earth, Geb, and diapers were prepared for it by the goddess of the sky, Nut, the divine mother caring for all of the gods in the form of the stars. The protective incantation was to be delivered over the bricks prepared for childbirth, by a person properly instructed for it.

Postnatal care of the mother

We know from the Westcar Papyrus, already quoted several times, that its heroine, the wife of the high priest of the supreme sun god Ra called Rudjdjedet, was purified after childbirth for fourteen days. For that time, the woman mainly remained in seclusion in the birth shelter, a light structure of posts and palm branches, the depiction of which can be found on several ostraca from the New Kingdom (fig. 53). In seclusion from the rest of the world, served by one of the young girls, the mother could devote herself to the newborn, breastfeed it, caress it, and comfort it. She also cared for her appearance and rested, so that she could later return refreshed to the everyday work of caring for the household, or as an assistant for her husband in raising domestic animals and working in the fields.

After the purification period, women carried their children everywhere with them, bound by a strip of cloth on their backs or astride on their side so that they could work. When the child demanded food, the mother squatted or knelt on the ground to be able to breastfeed it anywhere without embarrassment (fig. 54). For magical protection, mothers turned primarily to the goddess Isis, a diligent and experienced mother who, according to the myth, managed to protect her son Horus from all dangers and malicious enemies. The popularity of this goddess is manifested by the number of statues of Isis breastfeeding the young Horus, to which the various statuettes of mothers with an infant also refer. Breast milk was sometimes kept in ceramic vessels in the form of a kneeling Isis (fig. 55). Breast milk, particularly from a woman who had given birth to a boy, was considered a medicine for childhood intestinal disorders.

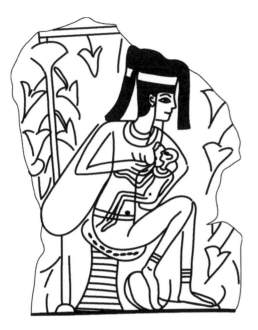

Fig. 53. An ostracon from Deir al-Medina bears a depiction of a young mother caring for her child in a childbirth shelter. It was sketched by one of the royal artists who lived in the village and who hewed and decorated the tombs in the royal Valley of the Kings. (Nineteenth/Twentieth Dynasties, British Museum in London [BM 8506], drawing: H. Vymazalová)

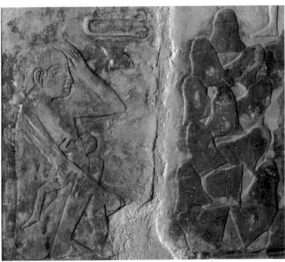

Fig. 54. A female baker with a nursing infant at her breast watches over the loaves of bread that are baking on the hearth. (Sixth Dynasty, tomb of Niankhkhnum and Khnumhotep at Saqqara, photo: M. Zemina)

The following group of cases from the Ebers Papyrus contains prescriptions that were to help the recovery of the uterus after childbirth. The healing preparations were composed of a number of herbal ingredients and plant juices; sometimes they also utilized honey or oil.

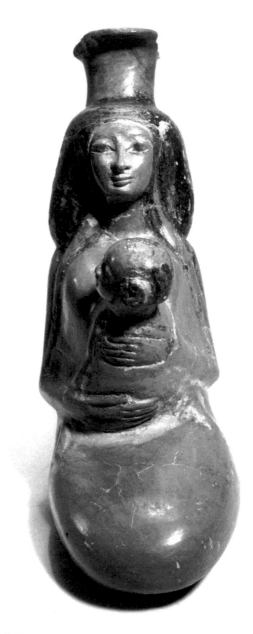

Fig. 55. Vessels in the shape of a woman with a child in her arms were very popular and were used to hold breast milk, which according to Egyptian beliefs had healing effects. (Eighteenth Dynasty, bpk/Egyptian Museum and Papyrus Collection, SMB/Margarete Büsing [14476])

Ebers 820: Cooling and contraction of the womb

This brief prescription describes a remedy that was probably to help against puerperal fever, which threatened mothers after childbirth. It comprised sorghum and yellow nutsedge mixed with oil, and the vagina was rinsed with this mixture. The final words "It is contraction of the uterus" indicate that the preparation could be applied to a woman even without fever, because it was simultaneously to help the contraction of the womb after childbirth, as in Cases Ebers 823–827 (see below).

Ebers 821: The same

Another prescription for the same problem was composed of a mixture of honey and hemp, which was applied by a douche to the woman's vagina.

Ebers 822: The same

Another remedy for the contraction of the uterus included a mixture of incense, celery, and milk, which was strained and applied by a douche to the woman's vagina.

Ebers 823: Contraction of the womb

This brief prescription describes a preparation which was to facilitate the contraction, that is, reduction in the size, of the emptied uterus after childbirth. It was composed of equal amounts of wild carrots, honey, juice from the pulp of carob pods, and milk, and this mixture was applied by a douche to the woman's vagina. Honey could in actuality be useful in this case. Its antibacterial and fungicidal effects could prevent an infection after childbirth and reduce possible swelling. According to Nunn (1996, 194), the preparation could serve not only for the acceleration of childbirth, but also for the expulsion of the placenta and return of the uterus to its normal size.

Ebers 824: The same

Another prescription for the same problem was composed only of a mixture of water and the drink *mesta*, which was applied by a douche to the woman's vagina.

Ebers 825: The same

Contraction of the uterus was supported also by potamogeton juice, which had astringent effects and was applied by a douche to the woman's vagina.

Ebers 826: The same

Another remedy for the contraction of the uterus was juice from the unknown *ketket* plant, which was applied by a douche to the woman's vagina.

Ebers 827: The same

Another prescription recommended juice from the unknown *niaia* plant, which was applied by a douche to the woman's vagina. This herb also appears in the preparations to induce childbirth or an abortion (see p. 175; Ebers 806).

Kahun 4: Swelling after childbirth

This is a case in which a large swelling formed in the woman's pubic region, perhaps after a difficult childbirth. From the description, Nunn (1996, 194) sees significant damage to the perineum, the ligament barrier between the vagina and the anus. The cure lies in the treatment of the private parts with 480 ml *(hin)* of fresh oil.

Kahun 6: Pain of the limbs and eye sockets

This case is very difficult to understand. It describes a woman suffering from pains in all of her limbs and in her eye sockets (they are the same manifestations as in Case Kahun 16, see p. 144). Griffith (1898, 7) believed that it is a starvation of the uterus, which is thirsty and is completely without nourishment—like a woman who has just given birth. Other translations (Collier and Quirke 2004) do not make much sense. It is likely that narrowing of the uterus could be connected with (or could be aggravated by) drinking beer after childbirth, because the text contains a command for the woman to abstain entirely from its consumption (Westendorf 1999, 414). The treatment was to be ensured by (oat) porridge with water consumed in the morning for several days.

Kahun 17: Bleeding

The case has not been preserved in its entirety, but it is relatively easy to understand. It concerns a woman who is bleeding from the uterus, from which the placenta has not yet come out. She also has headaches as well as pains in her mouth and palms. The diagnosis has not been preserved, but it could be a case of a late, in other words difficult, separation of the placenta or its parts from the uterine wall ("when everything does not come out of her"). The uterus is a muscular ligamentary sac, sufficiently solid and able to expand during the growth of the fetus. Its tearing, for example through a rough course of childbirth or local disruption of the blood circulation, occurs rarely. The treatment lies in the preparation of a clean place on the ground, where the woman is first seated on the dregs of sweet beer, to which squeezed dates are subsequently added. If even this does not help and the entire placenta does not come out of the body, the woman is to be given a boiled and cooled drink whose composition has not been preserved. If, however, blood with pus also comes out of the woman, it can be a sign of a more serious problem, most likely a complication in the form of an inflammation.

Ebers 789: Placenta
A group of cases in the Ebers Papyrus concerns the expulsion of the placenta. According to some interpretations of these cases, the word 'placenta' could also refer to the uterus; this would thus be a direct parallel to Case Ebers 795 (see below), but the first possibility seems more likely (see also Bardinet 1995, 225). This prescription described how to prepare a "cloth brick," or rather a pad soaked with a mixture of (beer) dregs and cedar sawdust, on which the woman was seated so that the medicine could act on her womb.

Ebers 790: The same
Another prescription for causing the expulsion of the placenta was intended to be applied on the womb and included clay reinforced with honey.

Ebers 791: The same
According to this prescription, beer dregs and unidentified dirt from a boat, perhaps sediments or mud, were used magically for the expulsion of the placenta. The woman was to drink this repulsive mixture in the dregs of excellent beer.

Ebers 792: The same
Another prescription recommends a mixture of ochre and myrrh, with which the abdomen of the woman was smeared, and a bandage dipped in myrrh was applied as well. Myrrh, the resin of the tree *Commiphora* that grows in Ethiopia, Somalia, and south Arabia, is recommended for external application in a number of medical papyri.

Ebers 793: The same
According to the title, this and the following case (Ebers 794) offer other prescriptions for the same problems. The description of the problems themselves, however, is missing in the text, and the medical procedure in these cases is based on magical methods, which were to be applied in the cases where other means did not help. The medicinal mixture, which included incense mixed with dried human feces, was intended for the fumigation of the sexual organs.

Ebers 794: The same

Another prescription after childbirth also included dried human feces. This time, however, they were to be ground in beer foam and the woman was to dip her fingers into this mixture and touch herself where it hurt.

Ebers 795: Returning the womb to its place

In this case, the uterus was to return to its place, but it is not clear from the text what the problems were. Most likely, it was the descent of a wandering uterus to its place, not the return of the uterus after childbirth, because the enlarged uterus, pregnant with the fetus, remains in place even after childbirth. The medical procedure included fumigation of the genitalia with a wax figurine of an ibis, which slowly melted above glowing coals. According to Egyptian ideas, the ibis was connected with regeneration.

Breasts

For the long period of breastfeeding, an Egyptian woman had to care for the cleanliness of her nipples to prevent their infection and thus not to threaten the health of her child. A certain group of cases in the Ebers Papyrus and the Papyrus Berlin 3038 are devoted to breast problems. The causes of these problems are not specified in most cases. Manifestations, however, include pains or swelling of the breasts and limbs. The treatment methods lie in

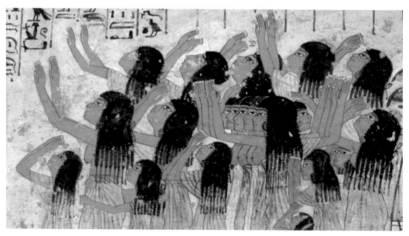

Fig. 56. Women in a funeral procession pour dust on their hair in a sign of mourning, and their eyes are full of tears. The older woman at the head of the procession has limp breasts, whereas the younger girls behind her are depicted with beautifully shaped, firm breasts. (Eighteenth Dynasty, tomb of Ramose [TT 55] in Sheikh Abd al-Qurna, photo: M. Zemina)

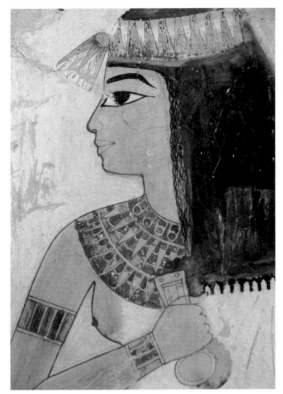

Fig. 57. The breasts were depicted without embarrassment, and in the reliefs and paintings they often project from the fine robes and hence emphasize the elegant figures of Egyptian women. (Eighteenth Dynasty, tomb of Nakht [TT 52] in Sheikh Abd al-Qurna, photo: M. Megahed)

smearing the breasts with a mixture of various herbal ingredients, honey, and minerals. Unfortunately, we do not yet know many of them, and it is thus difficult to evaluate the efficacy of the quoted means.

In the course of the menstrual cycle, the breasts react to the secretion of ovarian hormones. The feeling of tension, sometimes even pain, in the breasts is a component of premenstrual tension (pp. 140–41). In pregnancy, the front lobe of the pituitary gland releases the luteotropic or lactogenic hormone, prolactin, which maintains the viability of the corpus luteum in the ovary and stimulates it for the creation and release of progesterone. Along with estrogen, produced in the ovaries, it morphologically and functionally prepares the mammary glands before the end of the pregnancy for the production of breast milk, which it maintains for the entire period of breast-feeding (lactation).

The normal need for milk increases from childbirth to the tenth week, when it amounts to 900–950 grams per day. Its production is dependent not only on the sucking ability of the infant and the complete emptying of the breasts, but also on the mental state of the mother, who should live in happy contentment. A reduction of the amount of secreted milk (hypogalaxy) occurs in imperfectly developed or diseased breasts, in disorders of the overall health of the mother, or with poor breastfeeding technique. It can also be caused by the weak sucking of immature, particularly prematurely born, or ill infants (for example, with a cleft lip or a nasal catarrh).

The opposite case is the excessive production of milk. The Ebers Papyrus speaks of an illness called *gesu*. Most scholars do not translate this expression (Nunn 1996, 197; Bardinet 1995, 447) and do not comment on the given problems or treatment, but the word *gesu* in Egyptian means 'overflowing' (Hannig 1997, 907) and thus could have labeled the spontaneous flow of milk from overly full breasts, or painful swellings of full mammary glands. The recommended remedies were applied not only to the breasts but sometimes also to the pubic region.

Ebers 808: Falling of the breasts and overflowing of the breasts
According to the title of this case, it seems that this could have been a prescription against the deformation (dropping) of the breasts, probably influenced by maternity. The breasts were to be washed with the blood of a girl who had just begun to menstruate. In addition, the abdomen and thighs should be smeared to prevent "overflowing" of the breasts *(gesu)*, that is, their being too full or overflowing as a consequence of excessive milk production during lactation.

Ebers 809: Overflowing of the breasts
According to these instructions, dried swallow liver ground with a decoction of medicinal herbs also helped to avoid "overflowing" of the breasts *(gesu)*. The mixture was applied to the breasts, abdomen, and limbs of the patient.

Berlin 14: Swelling of the breasts and limbs
This case describes a preparation to limit swelling of the breasts and limbs, which was composed of wheat, pulp of carob pods, dates, date sourdough, and natron. The mixture was stirred and spread on painful breasts.

Berlin 15: The same
Another prescription for the same problems was a mixture from the pulp of carob pods, honey, and a mineral called the "great protection." The procedure was the same as in the previous case.

Berlin 16: The same

Another prescription describes a mixture of honey, salt, and the unidentified plants *tjun* and *ihu*. The method was the same as in the previous cases.

Ebers 810: Breast pain

This case describes a medical preparation for breast pain, whose cause is in no way specified. The magical mixture included the unknown mineral *hetem*, bull's bile, fly droppings, and ochre, and was used for smearing on the breasts for a period of four days.

Berlin 13: Breast pain

Only a small part of this case has been preserved, but apparently it is a preparation to drive away pains of the breasts. The prescription included honey and thyme.

Berlin 17: Breast pain

In this case, painful breasts were treated with bull's bile, fly droppings, and ochre. The painful breast was coated with the mixture.

Berlin 18: Breast pain

A prescription composed of natron and salt, which were mixed with honey and the pulp of carob pods, could also be applied to painful breasts. The ingredients are similar to those in Case Berlin 15 and could act osmotically and as an anti-inflammatory. The mixture was to be boiled and used for the repeated coating of the breast.

Ebers 811: Spell for the breast

The title of this case does not mention the precise purpose of the prescription, which for the most part is a magical incantation. The text of the incantation probably addresses the disease of the breast itself and calls on it not to empty itself, not to be eaten away, and not to bleed. Manifestations described in this way could testify to an inflammation or an ulcerous carcinoma of the breast, arising from the lactiferous ducts. This case was also interpreted as breast cancer by Nunn (1996, 197). The great pain connected with this illness is indicated by the comparison of the breast of the treated woman with the breast of the goddess Isis, which hurt her when she was giving birth to the god of the air, Shu, and the goddess of moisture, Tefnut (Janák 2005, 171, 174–75). The incantation was to be delivered over a roll of plant fibers that was rolled to the left and on which seven knots were made; it was to be placed on the affected spot on the woman's body.

Care of Children

The immense love of the ancient Egyptians for children is very apparent (Matiegková 1937; Feucht 1995) (fig. 59). The depictions on the walls of Egyptian tombs, on steles, and in numerous sculptures, capture small children with their parents as they enjoyed life on the fertile banks of the life-giving Nile. In the depictions, small children are usually naked, the smallest with a finger in his or her mouth, and their hair falls to one side in the so-called side-lock of youth. If children were depicted in the reliefs, paintings, or statues next to their parents, they sometimes preserved their childlike appearance, despite the fact that they may have already reached maturity (fig. 58).

The world of children was not exactly idyllic in the conditions of ancient Egyptian life. It is estimated that every second or third child died in infancy or childhood. With every month, the curve of mortality of nursing children below the age of three decreased. Nevertheless, around three years of age, with the weaning of children and the shift to artificial nourishment, it again rose somewhat, evidently as a consequence of an increase in intestinal infections (Strouhal and Bareš 1993, 71–72). There were many illnesses, and they affected a great percentage of the children. The skeletal remains prove frequent cases of growth arrest (the so-called Harris line), which emerge as a consequence of a longer illness or lack of adequate nourishment.

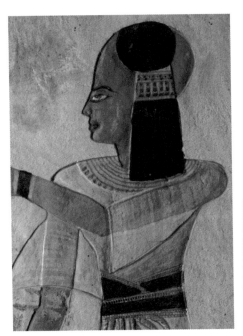

Fig. 58. Although the eldest son of King Ramesses III, Khaemwaset, lived to adulthood and held a high position, he was always depicted next to his father as a mere child. His hairstyle, the so-called sidelock of youth, was typical for children at the time of the New Kingdom. (Nineteenth Dynasty, tomb of Khaemwaset [QV 44] in the Valley of the Queens, photo: M. Megahed)

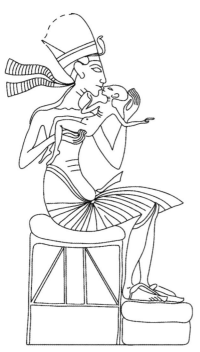

Fig. 59. The sovereign Akhenaten, who was famous for his daring reforms in religion and artistic style, is often depicted as a loving father. (Eighteenth Dynasty, Egyptian Museum in Berlin, drawing: H. Vymazalová after Wildung 1994, p. 24)

In the texts devoted to children's problems, medical science and magic intermingle. In newborns, the chance of survival was estimated, and magical protection in the form of amulets was made for them. Some cases describe the illnesses that could affect "a child or an adult." They concern disorders of urination, bronchitis, and various other infections.

The protection of children from diseases was to be ensured by preparations of herbal and mineral ingredients, but also by magic. Superstitious mothers cared for their children following the model of Isis, who with her powers protected the young Horus in the papyrus bushes, where they were both hiding from Seth. This form of the god Horus was called Harpakhered (literally 'Horus the Child,' in Greek Harpocrates), and the texts often contain allusions to diseases or problems to which the young Horus was exposed (Wilkinson 2003, 132; Janák 2005, 86). Isis, however, with her magical power, always managed to protect him, and through spells that the mothers recited over their sick children, the goddess protected them as well.

A comprehensive collection of the incantations, called the *Book for Mother and Child*, describes various methods of protection for the mother and her offspring. They are based upon invoking diverse deities and their abilities to protect various parts of the body and increase the effectiveness of the amulets prepared following the precisely defined methods. We find among the purely magical instructions several prescriptions from herbal ingredients, which were to help in illnesses of an unknown origin.

Tests of the viability of the newborn

Comparatively few of the children born had a real chance of survival. The mother and child were threatened predominantly by various infections, puerperal fever in the mothers and intestinal infection in the newborns, which were relatively frequent considering the poor hygienic conditions in ancient Egypt. Many children died within a few days after birth, but with every day, week, or month their chances of survival increased. Natural selection also screened out the weak or disabled individuals.

Children's tombs are much less frequent than we might expect. Sometimes the newborn child was buried with the mother if both died soon after childbirth. At other times, the children's bodies were placed in clay containers under the floor of the houses, or the parents buried them in the desert sands (fig. 60), often outside of official burial grounds.

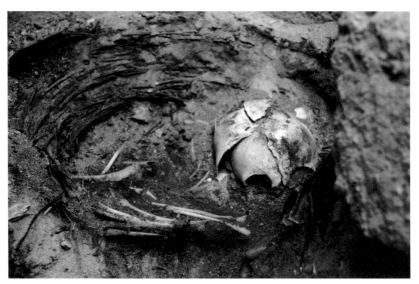

Fig. 60. The burial of a baby, discovered by the Czech mission in Egypt in March 2010, demonstrates the extreme love and pain of the bereaved parents. The small child was wrapped in linen, placed in a reed basket, and buried in a small circular tomb of mud brick. (Fifth Dynasty, Abusir, photo: H. Vymazalová)

Not every newborn revealed its craving for life with an energetic cry. If its cries were quiet, the face dull, and the body weak, it was necessary to use one of the tests of its viability. The prognoses of the survival of a newborn child were based on superstitions and surprisingly did not take note of its physical state at all. The hope of survival was to be increased by the use of special amulets and magical incantations.

Ebers 838: Prognosis of survival
This case describes how to determine the chances of survival in a newborn child. The method is based on what sound the child makes. If it sounds like "*ny*," the baby should survive; if, however, the child says something like "*embi*," it will die. This method is, naturally, nonsensical.

Ebers 839: Prognosis of survival
Another method for determining a newborn who should not survive claims that a newborn will not survive if it cries loudly or if it turns its face downward. It is not clear whether these are supposed to be the first reactions of the child after birth, or whether the child should be observed for a longer time, but undoubtedly it is also a nonsensical test.

Ramesseum IV.C ll. 15–16: Protection of a newborn
The case describes the way to make an amulet that should protect the baby immediately after its birth. Unfortunately, only a small part of the text has been preserved, which as an ingredient mentions a piece of the infant's first stool (meconium) and which undoubtedly belongs to the realm of magic.

Ramesseum IV.C ll. 17–24: Prognosis of survival, protection of a newborn
This relatively detailed case describes another way to recognize whether the newborn baby will survive. Parts of its placenta were to be mixed with milk and given to the baby to drink. The newborn was to die if it vomited this mixture. If it swallowed the milk without any consequences, it showed the ability to survive. The prescription is followed by an incantation, which was to ensure magically the protection of the mother during childbirth (see above on p. 173).

Ramesseum IV.C ll. 25–28: Probably the same
This case has been preserved only in part, but we can judge that it is again a magical spell accompanying the production of a protective amulet for the child. The text has not been preserved in its entirety, but it mentions a number of significant gods, whose power was to benefit the newborn. The god

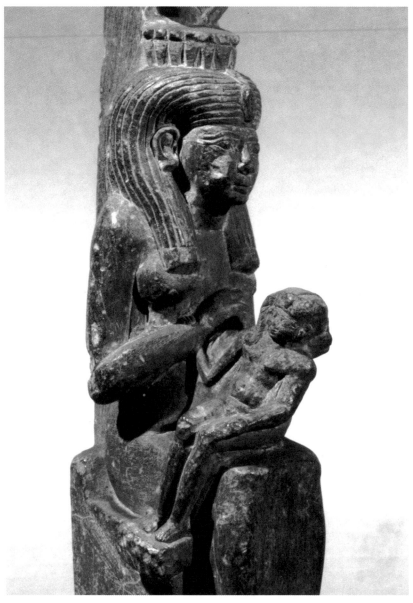

Fig. 61. The goddess Isis, breastfeeding the child god Horus, was often called upon for help by Egyptian mothers. Her magical power could protect children and mothers. Isis and Horus comprise an archetype of the Virgin Mary with Baby Jesus in her arms. (Late Period, Egyptian Museum, Cairo [JE 39282], photo: M. Zemina)

Hemen was able to ensure the destruction of enemies (Janák 2005, 73), and the goddesses Isis and Nephthys, related to him, also provided protection. Those further invoked include the god of the air, Shu; the goddess of the moisture of the air, Tefnut; the god of the earth, Geb; and the god of the underworld, Osiris. The rest of the text is not entirely clear, but it refers to the god Ha, who was an important protector from all types of danger (Wilkinson 2003, 106; Janák 2005, 60). The end of the text is unclear.

Book for Mother and Child V: Protection during childbirth and protection of a newborn child

This purely magical spell was to be delivered during childbirth so that it would be free of problems and the child would be protected from evil forces. The incantation invokes the protective goddesses Isis and Nephthys and is to banish all possible dangers that could harm the newborn. In the conclusion, a guide for the production of a protective amulet for the child has been added in red ink.

Breastfeeding and breast milk

As *The Maxims of Ani* mentions in the part devoted to family life and the relation to one's mother, ancient Egyptian women could breastfeed their children for as long as three years: "When you were born after your months, she was yet yoked (to you), her breast in your mouth for three years. As you grew and your excrement became disgusting, she was not disgusted, saying: What shall I do!" (Lichtheim 1976, 141).

During that long period of breastfeeding, women were more or less protected hormonally from another conception. The nourishment of breast milk also had an influence on the immunity of the infants to ailments, because it contained the mother's antibodies.

The hiring of wet nurses was widespread in ancient Egypt; in particular, women from the higher social classes did this, even if they themselves could breastfeed. The parents of a child concluded a written agreement with the wet nurse, setting out the rights and responsibilities of both parties involved. A very close bond often developed between the wet nurse and the child, and royal wet nurses could enjoy a significant position and influence at the royal court. Egyptians, moreover, believed that the transmission of breast milk created a certain relationship between children who were breastfed by the same woman. This idea has been maintained in Egypt to this day, and even in the Qur'an, the holy book of Islam, we find a ban on concluding marriages between a man and his wet nurse or milk (foster) sister (Qur'an 4:23).

The transmission of milk also formed a part of the royal ideological depictions on the walls of Egyptian temples. Here, the sovereigns often boasted that they drank the milk of some of the goddesses, predominantly of Isis. The goddess is sometimes depicted in the form of a celestial cow, and the ruler is kneeling under her and drinking directly from her udder (fig. 62). According to Egyptian ideas, in this way the royal child acquired divine power, supporting his claim to the throne and his monarchical abilities.

Difficulties with breastfeeding are the topic of one case in the Ramesseum Papyrus and are treated with the aid of a magical incantation. Several of the cases contained in the Ebers Papyrus deal with breast milk. Its quality was important for infants to thrive and be protected from digestive problems. The quality of the milk was judged based on its characteristic smell, and one case also provides a prescription for ensuring a sufficient amount of milk.

Great significance was ascribed to the breast milk of a woman who had given birth to a boy. It was considered to be a medicine and stored in vessels in the shape of the seated goddess Isis holding her son Horus. It was used to treat a cough in infants, and intestinal problems and eye diseases in children and adults.

Three cases contained on the fragments of the Ramesseum papyri mention thirst afflicting an infant. They concern either a declining production of

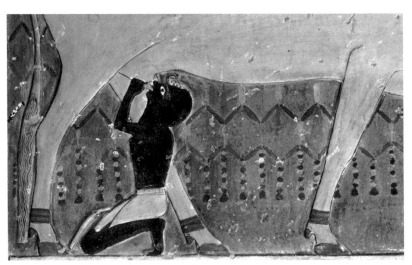

Fig. 62. Queen Hatshepsut sucks milk from the goddess Hathor, who takes the form of a divine cow. The golden color of the cow's body represents divinity, whereas the queen's skin is dark, symbolizing revival and renewal. (Eighteenth Dynasty, Hatshepsut's Chapel, Egyptian Museum, Cairo [JE 38575], photo: S. Vannini)

breast milk, or a child for which breastfeeding was complemented with mashed food so that the mother could gradually wean it.

Ramesseum III.B ll. 10–11: Problems with breastfeeding
This case deals with a child who refuses to drink milk from its mother's breast. Unfortunately, the incantation has been only partially preserved, referring to the gods Horus and Seth and the ability to swallow and bite.

Ebers 788: Deteriorated milk
The quality of breast milk was determined by smell. If it smelled like fish, it was not in order.

Ebers 796: Excellent milk
In this case, the smell of good breast milk was compared to the smell of earth almonds.

Ebers 836: The formation of milk
The method described in this case was to aid a breastfeeding woman or wet nurse caring for a baby to produce enough breast milk. Her back was to be rubbed with oil with the soft-cooked spine of the Nile perch.

Ramesseum III.A l. 9: Thirst
Only the title of this case has been preserved, which mentions quenching thirst in a child. The prescription has, however, been destroyed.

Ramesseum III.B ll. 14–17: Thirst
This case begins with a magical incantation that was to help against thirst in infants. The text is full of magical symbolism. Thirst is to be removed by the god Agebuer, whose name means 'Great Flood' and who was the god of abundance (Janák 2005, 17–18). In addition, the mention of the breast of the goddess Hesat, who is to feed the infant, is worth attention. Hesat was connected with motherhood and the donation of milk and had the appearance of a wild cow (Wilkinson 2003, 173–74). Osiris's spring symbolizes the Nile, upon which the subsistence of all of the population of the Nile Valley and Delta depended. All of these components of the incantation expressed the wish that the infant would always have enough food. The last part of the text is unfortunately destroyed, so we do not know the precise method of applying the magical incantation; a protective amulet might also have been made during the recitation.

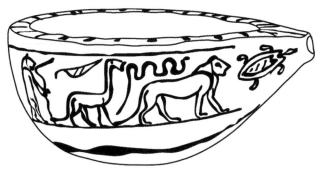

Fig. 63. A small bowl for feeding breast milk to the infant is decorated with protective idols in the form of animals. (Twelfth Dynasty, Metropolitan Museum of Art, New York, drawing: H. Vymazalová after Allen 2005, 31)

Ramesseum III.B ll. 19–20: Thirst

This case was to quench the thirst of a child as well as an adult. The ingredients of the healing mixture, which have not been preserved in the text, were to be left in water overnight according the described method, and after straining, 480 ml *(hin)* were given to the child (or adult) to drink.

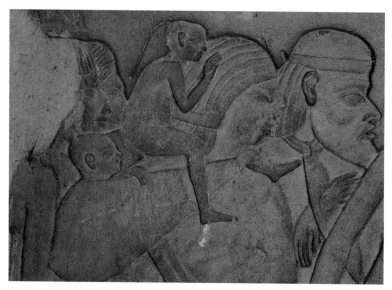

Fig. 64. In the procession of Asian captives, one of the women carries her two children. One is hanging in a bag tied to her back; the other child is sitting on her shoulders. (Eighteenth Dynasty, tomb of Horemheb at Saqqara, photo: M. Megahed)

Children's diseases

Ancient Egyptian children, particularly infants and toddlers, were threatened by a wide range of diseases. The most prevalent of these were diseases of the digestive tract, parasitic disease, and infections of childhood, but there was no lack of tuberculosis, rheumatism, avitaminosis, anemia, and many other sicknesses.

Testimony on the presence of a wide range of illnesses is provided by the archaeological surveys of cemeteries and detailed paleopathological analyses of the skeletal finds or mummies, examined with modern imaging technology. Burials from the Late, Ptolemaic, and Roman Periods, investigated by the Czech archaeological expedition at the burial grounds around the mastaba of Ptahshepses in Abusir, prove that a very high-risk time in the life of a child was age three to four, when the mother stopped breastfeeding. The transition to a normal diet without supplementation in the form of breast milk could have caused an increase in intestinal infections, and as a consequence, increased mortality (Strouhal and Bareš 1993, 71–72).

Children did not evade injuries either. Naturally, the medical papyri do not contain the names of the diseases that we know today, because the currently used terminology of nosological units (diseases with a known cause and mechanism of emergence) was not introduced until the last two centuries. The Egyptian texts list only the names of the symptoms, such as fever, cough, pain, or special terms labeling illnesses whose translation is not yet clear. In such cases, it is difficult to determine the nature of the disease, and not even the recommended treatment usually brings relief, since it is often based mainly on magical activities. Magic here compensates for the lack of knowledge of the causes of the illnesses.

The illnesses mentioned in the texts include *baa*, which appears in infants and is connected with the acceptance of breast milk. We do not know the characteristics of this problem; most likely it was an internal ailment whose cause was not apparent to Egyptian physicians. It might have been flatulence (Barns 1956, 22), which can give infants a very hard time, but according to the incantation in one of the Ramesseum Papyri, it could have been a more serious infection. Three of the recommended preparations were liquid, which is not surprising for infants.

Ramesseum III.B ll. 20–23: The illness *baa*

The medicinal treatment for *baa* relied only on a spell and the magical power of an amulet of acacia fibers, whose production it describes. The spell is almost incomprehensible, but it contains an interesting reference to a name. The invocation "Do not say my name" is connected with the ancient Egyptian idea that knowledge of the name gave power over the fate of its bearer. By concealing the real name, the mother hence ensured protection of her child.

Ramesseum III.B ll. 23–34: The illness *baa*

This case is composed of a very long incantation. The beginning of the text has been destroyed, but the problems that affected the child are apparent from the spell that follows. According to it, Horus, son of the goddess Isis, drank not only breast milk from her breast, but also the disease *baa*, which exhausted him, caused his lips to turn blue (a blood-circulation disorder), and made his knees buckle (made walking impossible). The "evil substance," perhaps an infection, hence came from Isis's breasts.

The incantation refers to the reaction of Isis when the young Horus became ill. The goddess sought counsel from her mother, the goddess of the sky Nut, who according to Egyptian ideas swallowed the sun every evening and gave birth to it again every morning. For her eternally regenerative role, she was connected also with Hathor (Wilkinson 2003, 160–63; Janák 2005, 131–32). According to the advice recommended in the text, the illness *baa* was to be transferred to a small swallow—it was most likely a small statue or amulet in the shape of a baby swallow, not a real bird. The small swallow's eyes were to be painted with galena, and at the same time a protective amulet was to be made for the child, braided from straw by the woman who had given birth to the child in question. The nestling of the swallow refers to the baby.

Book for Mother and Child O: The illness *baa*

This magical incantation is intended for a breastfeeding woman and her child, and is to help against the illness *baa*. It hence confirms the connection between breast milk and this illness. According to the text, the lamentation of the mother penetrated all the way to Duat, the place where the gods lived. The incantation mentions a whole range of protective gods, including the sun god Ra, the crocodile god Sobek, and the protective goddess Tayet. The child itself is compared to Horus, a divine child enjoying the protection of powerful gods. When delivering these words, a protective amulet, which is to be hung on the child's neck, is also to be prepared.

Book for Mother and Child H: The illness *baa*

Other cases described in the same text contain prescriptions for treating the illness *baa*. According to this case, a breastfeeding woman should drink a mixture from the fruits of the sycamore, fresh dates, a part of the castor oil plant, hemp, fibers of the *debyt* plant, and the drink *mesta*.

Book for Mother and Child I: The illness *baa*

Another prescription for the same problems recommends a mixture of papyrus bolls, earth almonds, and breast milk. The child was to drink 480 ml *(hin)* of this so that its sleep would be uninterrupted.

Book for Mother and Child K: The illness *baa*

Another prescription for the same problems suggests the grinding of twigs of an unidentified plant *nebu* in 480 ml *(hin)* of water; this preparation is given to the child to drink.

Ebers 782: Constant crying

For a child who screamed too much because of flatulence, pains, or sleeplessness, a decoction of poppy seeds and fly droppings scraped from the wall was prepared. Poppy seeds must have been an effective means for reliably inducing sleep, although it could become dangerous in longer-term application because of its opiate content. The period of administration was therefore limited to four days. Fly droppings were a magical additive. The explanatory note in the conclusion of the case, which clarifies the definition of an excessive scream, is interesting. It is reminiscent of the explanatory notes from the Edwin Smith Surgical Papyrus (see chapter 3).

Berlin 30: Cough

This case describes a medicine for a cough (in Egyptian *sery*). The child was to be given a mixture of 480 ml *(hin)* of milk with mashed dates. The warm and date-sweetened milk successfully helped moderate the cough by dissolving mucus.

Ebers 835: The illness *idju*

The problems described in this case are labeled with the Egyptian expression *idju*, whose meaning we unfortunately do not know. The symptoms are not described in the text; the healing mixture included unknown herbal ingredients.

Ramesseum IV.C ll. 6–7: The illness *neshu*

Only a small part of this case has been preserved. The problems that the child suffered from were called *neshu*, which means 'flowing' or 'leakage' (Hannig 1997, 434), but a precise description of these problems has not been preserved in the text. The name of the disease is reminiscent of urinary incontinence. The recommended medicinal drink included henbane, barley, an herbal decoction, and other ingredients.

Book for Mother and Child A: The illness *neshu*

Another case against the illness *neshu* describes a magical method by which beads of various colors produced from diverse stones are enchanted. These beads are then to be threaded on a string of yarn and given to the child as a protective amulet.

Book for Mother and Child E: The illness *neshu*

This lovely magical spell was also to aid against the illness *neshu*, which affected all of the limbs of the child. It is the longest incantation that has been preserved, where the child is compared to Horus and thus is assured the protection of the gods, primarily Isis.

Further in the text, the disease itself is addressed and called upon to leave all of the parts of the child's body alone and not to cause any harm to them. Each named part of the body was thus to acquire protection through this incantation. It proceeds from the head all the way to the soles of the feet, although in a somewhat jumbled order, from the crown of the head and forehead, through the eyebrows, eyes, nose, chest, mouth, vertebrae, throat, tongue, lips, chin, temples, ears, neck, shoulders, arms, fingers, bosom, skin, abdomen, navel, pubic region, penis, pelvis, back, rectum, buttocks, legs, knee, ankles, and feet, including the soles. What is medically interesting are the magical pieces

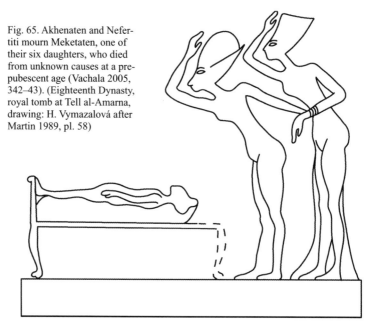

Fig. 65. Akhenaten and Nefertiti mourn Meketaten, one of their six daughters, who died from unknown causes at a prepubescent age (Vachala 2005, 342–43). (Eighteenth Dynasty, royal tomb at Tell al-Amarna, drawing: H. Vymazalová after Martin 1989, pl. 58)

of advice concerning what needs to be avoided, for instance defecating on the crown of the head, warping the forehead, making the eyebrows fall out, eye ailments (particularly amblyopia), nose maladies, hitting the throat, deafness, constriction of the neck, making the bosom hang down, intertrigo or chafing of the penis, a bad odor from the pelvis, hemorrhoids in the rectum, or paralysis of the knees. Furthermore, the mouth is to be prevented from having secrets, and the pubic region is to be prevented from having anything that the gods forbade.

Less comprehensible, although poetically beautiful, are the epithets comparing the breasts to the breasts of Hathor, the tongue to a snake from a cave, the chin to the tail of a duck, the shoulders to falcons, the navel to the morning star, and so on.

Book for Mother and Child L: The illness *sesemy*

This case does not describe the problems that the child suffers from, and the words of the magical spell indicate only a little of their nature. It could be, for example, an eye disease or chill in connection with the sun and heat. The incantation mentions the goddesses Sekhmet, Hathor, and Wadjet, who represent Ra's 'solar' eye, a symbol of power and protection.

The epithet "Great" probably refers to the god of the sun Ra, whose eye is to replace the injured eye of the god Horus (represented by the patient), which was hurt in a savage mythical struggle between Horus and his adversary Seth.

For the child, a protective amulet is produced at the same time from the bones of a mouse that the child or the mother has eaten, depending on whether the child is able to eat on its own or drinks breast milk.

Book for Mother and Child B: The disease *temyt*

The nature of the disease *temyt* is not entirely clear. It might have been a skin disease caused by a demon (Hannig 1997, 932), but according to the wording of this magical incantation, *temyt* was felt in the bones and blood vessels, could cause abdominal pain, and was to be driven out of the head and all of the limbs. Protection was to be ensured by calling on the god Ra and the goddesses Isis and Nephthys (fig. 66). The god Khnum, who created people on a potter's wheel, is also mentioned.

Book for Mother and Child C: The disease *temyt*

Another unclear spell, perhaps intended to fight the same illness, addresses and intimidates the disease itself, or the demon that allegedly caused it. Along with the incantation, a medicine or an amulet was to be made of yellow sweet clover, onion, honey, a piece of fabric, the spine of the Nile perch, and the tail

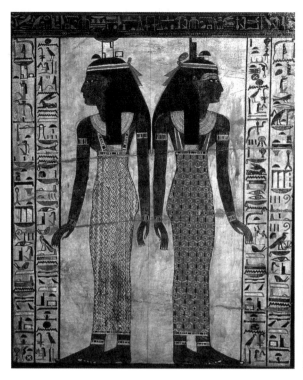

Fig. 66. The goddesses Isis and Nephthys (left), divine sisters and protectors of women and children. (Nineteenth Dynasty, Egyptian Museum, Cairo [JE 27302], photo: M. Zemina)

of the sacred fish *abedju*, which had great mythological importance because it accompanied the barque of the sun god and announced the nearness of his arch enemy Apophis, the representative of evil (Wilkinson 2003, 221–23; Janák 2005, 30–31).

Book for Mother and Child D: Protective incantation

The spell intended for the expulsion of an unknown disease compares this illness to Asian and Nubian women coming from inhospitable regions beyond Egypt. The incantation calls on it to leave the child through his vomit, urine, mucus, or sweat. Protection for the child is to be ensured by the goddess Isis, as she ensured it for her son Horus.

Book for Mother and Child M: Protective incantation and amulet

The spells that are recorded in the second half of this papyrus (Berlin 3027) do not describe or mention any particular health problems. They probably served as preventive, protective incantations for the child and its mother during childbirth and afterward.

This quite damaged incantation was to be delivered while placing a hand on the child. The text is hard to understand; it mentions the cobra goddess Iaret and the god of mummification Anubis, Isis's protector. There is also a discussion of the sacred fish *adju* (perhaps striped mullet from the Mugilidae family), with a warning to those who do not eat its meat. Moreover, a protective amulet is to be made from a part of this fish.

Book for Mother and Child N: Protective incantation and amulet
This spell is very hard to understand, and we cannot grasp the meaning of some passages at all. For the child's protection, the text summons the goddess Hathor, a guardian connected with maternity (Wilkinson 2003, 139–45), who is to help against the harmful powers of the dead or demons. This is followed by instructions for the production of a protective amulet.

Book for Mother and Child P: Protective incantation and amulet
In this spell, the child is compared to a nestling that is alone and helpless, entirely defenseless, and exposed to danger from harmful forces. The incantation is delivered during the production of the amulet.

Book for Mother and Child Q–T: Protective incantation
These four spells following consecutively in the text are almost identical. They are texts that were to be delivered over a child at sunrise and sunset, to invoke the protection of the gods for it. The crucial role here is played by Ra, the creator and lord of all (Wilkinson 2003, 205–209). The names of the child and its mother were to be added in the relevant passages to personalize the protection.

Book for Mother and Child U: Protective incantation
This gorgeous and poetic spell was to ensure protection of the child by comparing the individual parts of the body to the corresponding parts of the bodies of important gods. This was done systematically from the head through the body, upper limbs, and internal organs all the way to the lower limbs.

Problems with urination and defecation
In infants and toddlers, problems with urination (dysuria) could appear. With boys, they may be caused by narrowing of the foreskin opening (phimosis), which can be either congenital or acquired and non-inflammatory (after an injury), or inflammatory (in an infection of the glans and inner side of the foreskin). In boys and girls, problems with urination may be caused by an infection of the urethra and/or bladder. Another problem is bedwetting (enuresis),

which sometimes continues even after the third year of a child's life. It is usually caused by anxiety neurosis, but also by neglect in childrearing.

Even more frequently, small children have problems with defecation. They take the form of either obstipation caused by various intestinal diseases or dietary imbalances, or diarrhea resulting from intestinal infections or eating food that is too fatty or spicy.

Ebers 262: Urination
This case describes a prescription for helping a child to pass urine. Its belly was to be smeared with a mixture of oil with a papyrus scroll, boiled to mush. If the recommended mixture was to be applied warm, the massage could release the contraction of the sphincter of the bladder and actually ease urination for the child.

Ebers 272 bis: Urination
This prescription was to ensure that the infant urinated normally. The medicinal potion of the pith from a reed, sweet beer, and the unknown drink *khawy* was to be drunk by the woman, who thus passed on the effect of the medicine to her child through her breast milk.

Ebers 273: Bedwetting
A help against bedwetting was to be faience balls, which an older child was to swallow and an infant given to drink with the milk of his wet nurse. The treatment lasted for four days. The faience balls could work 'magically' (that is, by suggestion) on the older child, but they probably did not help the infants.

Ramesseum IV.C ll. 12–15: Evacuation
This case describes a magical spell which, with Isis's assistance, was to cure a child of problems with the evacuation of feces. How precisely to proceed during the incantation has not been preserved in the text. The spell and green bead laid on the belly activate the magical effect; "painful excrement" indicates that it might have been constipation.

Ramesseum III.A ll. 1–2: Constipation
This case has not been preserved in its entirety, and its wording is not completely clear. The child may have suffered from constipation. The medicine in this case was the mineral "great protection," which was likely pulverized and mixed with a liquid to enable the child to drink it.

Ramesseum III.A ll. 30–31: Urination

The prescription from this case was intended to ensure normal urination. The mixture comprised reed, beer, and the sediments from the drink *khawy*, which might have been an herbal beverage. The ingredients were to be drunk after mixing; the beer ensured the diuretic effect of the medicine. The preparation was intended for a child as well as for an adult, but the method of application differed.

Ramesseum III.B ll. 12–14: Fragment of a case

The beginning of this case has not been preserved, and thus neither the cause of the problem nor its manifestations are known. The text contains the rest of a prescription from salt and other ingredients, as well as a magical incantation to be recited during the production of the amulet. The method is intended for a child as well as an adult.

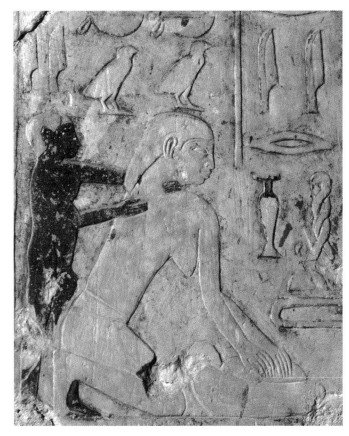

Fig. 67. A small child holds on to its mother, who is grinding grain for preparing bread. (Sixth Dynasty, tomb of Niankhkhnum and Khnumhotep at Saqqara, photo: M. Zemina)

BRIEF OVERVIEW OF THE HISTORY OF ANCIENT EGYPT

Today, we divide the history of ancient Egypt into several periods that reflect the greater or lesser stability of the state. We provide a brief characterization and selected monuments for the individual dynasties. The data shown are approximate; only the events in the first millennium BC can be dated with certainty (following Verner, Bareš, and Vachala 1998).

Predynastic Period (about 4500–3150 BC)
Earlier, Middle, Later
Dynasty Zero: process of the unification of Egypt

Archaic Period (about 3150–2700 BC)
First Dynasty (about 3150–2930 BC)
Second Dynasty (about 2930–2700 BC)

Old Kingdom (about 2700–2180 BC)
Third Dynasty (about 2700–2630 BC): step pyramids (Djoser's in Saqqara)
Fourth Dynasty (about 2630–2510 BC): centralized state; large pyramids at Meidum, Dahshur, Giza
Fifth Dynasty (about 2510–2365 BC): more modest pyramids in Abusir and Saqqara; sun temples
Sixth Dynasty (about 2365–2180 BC): pyramids in Saqqara; Pyramid Texts; gradual breakdown of the state structure

First Intermediate Period (about 2180–1994 BC)

Seventh Dynasty (about 2180–2170 BC): weakening of central power; development of local traditions

Eighth Dynasty (about 2170–2160 BC): development of local traditions

Ninth and Tenth Dynasties (about 2160–2137 BC): sovereigns residing in Herakleopolis

Eleventh Dynasty (about 2137–1994 BC): sovereigns residing in Thebes; unification of Egypt

Middle Kingdom (about 1994–1797 BC)

Twelfth Dynasty (about 1994–1797 BC): pyramids in Saqqara, Dahshur, Lisht, Lahun, Hawara

Second Intermediate Period (about 1797–1543 BC)

Thirteenth Dynasty (about 1797–1634 BC): gradual breakdown of central power

Fourteenth Dynasty: less significant rulers reigning in the Delta

Fifteenth Dynasty (about 1634–1526 BC): Hyksos sovereigns ruling in the northern part of the land

Sixteenth Dynasty: vassals of the Hyksos

Seventeenth Dynasty (about 1634–1543 BC): rulers residing in Thebes and reigning only in the southern part of the land; unification of Egypt and expulsion of the Hyksos

New Kingdom (about 1543–1078 BC)

Eighteenth Dynasty (about 1543–1292 BC): expansive policy and flowering of diplomacy; cliff tombs in the Valley of the Kings; large temple complexes

Nineteenth Dynasty (about 1292–1186 BC): military expeditions; extensive building activity

Twentieth Dynasty (about 1188–1078 BC): gradual breakdown of central power

Third Intermediate Period (about 1078–715 BC)

Twenty-first Dynasty (about 1078–945 BC): division of power between the rulers and the high priests

Twenty-second Dynasty (945–715 BC): rulers of Libyan origin in Tanis and Bubastis

Twenty-third Dynasty (818–715 BC): rulers of Libyan origin in Leontopolis

Twenty-fourth Dynasty (728/727–720 BC): independent ruler in the western part of the Delta

Late Period (715–305 BC)

Twenty-fifth Dynasty (745–664 BC): rulers from Nubia

Twenty-sixth Dynasty (665–525 BC): return to Egyptian traditions; the so-called Saite Renaissance; Greek communities in Egypt

Twenty-seventh Dynasty (525–404 BC): the first Persian rule

Twenty-eighth Dynasty (404–399 BC): short reign of the ruler Amenirdis

Twenty-ninth Dynasty (399–380 BC): shorter reigns by the rulers, originally the military commanders

Thirtieth dynasty (380–343 BC): prosperity of the land; building on the traditions from the period of the Saite rulers; battles for the independence of Egypt

Thirty-first Dynasty (343–332 BC): second Persian rule

Alexander the Great and other Greek rulers, Wars of the Diadochi (332–305 BC)

Ptolemaic Period (305–30 BC)

Great influence of Greece on Egyptian culture; Alexandria the center of education

Roman Period (30 BC–AD 395)

Byzantine Period (AD 395–640)

AD 640: conquest of Egypt by Arabs

BIBLIOGRAPHY

Allen, J.P. 2005. *The Art of Medicine in Ancient Egypt*. New York: Metropolitan Museum of Art.

Assmann, J. 1995. *Ma'at: Gerechtigkeit und Unsterblichkeit im Alten Ägypten*. Munich: C.H. Beck.

Bardinet, T. 1995. *Les papyrus médicaux de l'Égypte pharaonique. Traduction intégrale et commentaire*. Paris: Fayard.

Barns, J.W.B. 1956. *Five Ramesseum Papyri*. Oxford: Oxford University Press.

Bietak, M., and E. Strouhal. 1974. "Die Todesumstände des Pharaons Seqenenre."*Annalen des Naturhistorischen Museums Wien* 78: 29–52.

Bisset, N.G., J.G. Bruhn, S. Curto, B. Holmstedt, B.U. Nyman, and M.H. Zenk. 1994. "Was Opium Known in 18th Dynasty Ancient Egypt? An Examination of Materials from the Tomb of the Chief Royal Architect Kha." *Ethnopharmacology* 41: 99–114.

Brawarski, A. 2001. "Die Fälle 1–8 des Papyrus Edwin Smith ('Schädelhirntraumafälle')." *Studien zur altägyptischen Kultur* 29: 7–39.

———. 2004. "Die Würbelsäulenverletzungen des Papyrus Edwin Smith (Fall 29–33)." *Studien zur altägyptischen Kultur* 32: 59–80.

Breasted, J.H. 1930. *The Edwin Smith Surgical Papyrus*. Chicago: University of Chicago Press.

Brugsch, H. 1863. *Recueil des monuments égyptiens. Deuxième partie*. Leipzig: J.C. Hinrichs.

Bryan, C.P. 1930. *The Papyrus Ebers*. London: Geoffrey Bless.

Capel, A.K., and G.E. Markoe. 1996. *Mistress of the House, Mistress of Heaven: Women in Ancient Egypt*. New York: Hudson Hills Press.

Celsus, A.C. 1906. *Über die Arzneiwissenschaft in acht Büchern [De medicina]*. Translated by W. Frieboes. Braunschweig: Viewegh und Sohn.

Chapman, P.H. 1992. "Case Seven of the Smith Surgical Papyrus: The Meaning of *tp3w*." *Journal of the American Research Center in Egypt* 29: 35–42.

Collier, M., and S. Quirke. 2004. *The UCL Lahun Papyri: Religious, Literary, Legal, Mathematical, and Medical*. BAR International Series 1209. Oxford: Archaeopress.

Dastugue, J. 1967. "Pathologie des crânes d'Aksha." In *Aksha III. La population du cimetière méroïtique*, by M.C. Chamla, 157–71. Paris: Firmin Didot.

————. 1975. "Pathologie des hommes épipaléolithiques d'Afalou-Bou-Rhummel (Algérie)." *L'Anthropologie* 77: 63–92.

David, R., ed. 2008. *Egyptian Mummies and Modern Science*. Cambridge: Cambridge University Press.

Davies, N. de Garis. 1927. *Two Ramesside Tombs at Thebes*. New York: Metropolitan Museum of Art.

Dawson, W.R. 1932. "Studies in the Egyptian Medical Texts." *Journal of Egyptian Archaeology* 18: 150–54.

————. 1933. "Studies in the Egyptian Medical Texts II." *Journal of Egyptian Archaeology* 19: 133–37.

————. 1934a. "Studies in the Egyptian Medical Texts III." *Journal of Egyptian Archaeology* 20: 41–46.

————. 1934b. "Studies in the Egyptian Medical Texts IV." *Journal of Egyptian Archaeology* 20: 185–88.

————. 1935. "Studies in the Egyptian Medical Texts V." *Journal of Egyptian Archaeology* 21: 37–40.

Dawson, W.R., E.P. Uphill, and M.L. Bierbrier. 1995. *Who Was Who in Egyptology*. 3rd ed. London: Egypt Exploration Society.

Diodorus of Sicily. 1933. *Bibliotheca Historica 1, Book I–II*. London: William Heinemann.

Ebbell, B. 1928. "Der chirurgische Teil des Papyrus Ebers." *Acta Orientalia* 7: 1–47.

————. 1937. *The Papyrus Ebers: The Greatest Egyptian Medical Document*. Copenhagen: Levin & Munksgaard.

————. 1939. *Die altägyptische Chirurgie. Die chirurgischen Abschnitte der Papyrus E. Smith und Papyrus Ebers*. Skrifter utgitt av det Norske Videnskaps-Akademi i Oslo. II. Hist-Filos. Klasse No. 2. Oslo: Dybward.

Ebeid, N.I. 1999. *Egyptian Medicine in the Days of the Pharaohs*. Cairo: General Egyptian Book Organization.

Ebers, G.M. 1875. *Papyros Ebers: das hermetische Buch über die Arzeneimittel der alten Ägypter in hieratischer Schrift I–II*. Leipzig: Engelmann.

Erman, A. 1890. *Die Märchen des Papyrus Westcar I–II*. Mitteilungen aus den Orientalischen Sammlungen VI. W. Berlin: Spemann.

———. 1901. *Zaubersprüche für Mutter und Kind aus dem Papyrus 3027 des Berliner Museums*. Berlin: Königliche Akademie der Wissenschaften.

Estes, J.W. 1989. *The Medical Skills of Ancient Egypt*. Canton, MA: Science History Publications U.S.A.

Faied, M. El-Hoseiny. 2006. *Ancient Egyptian Medicine*. Cairo.

Feucht, E. 1995. *Das Kind im Alten Ägypten*. Frankfurt: Campus Verlag.

Firth, C.M. 1915. *The Archaeological Survey of Nubia. Report for 1909–1910*. Cairo: Government Press.

Frey, E.F. 1985–86. "The Earliest Medical Texts." *Clio Medica* 20, nos. 1–4: 79–90.

Gardiner, A.H. 1935. *Hieratic Papyri in the British Museum*. London: British Museum.

———. 1955. *The Ramesseum Papyri*. Oxford: Oxford University Press.

Germer, R. 1979. "Untersuchung über Arzneimittelpflanzen im Alten Ägypten." Doctoral diss., Universität Hamburg.

———. 2002. *Die Heilpflanzen der Ägypter*. Düsseldorf: Artemis.

———. 2008. *Handbuch der altägyptischen Heilpflanzen*. Philippika. Marburger altertumskundliche Abhandlungen 21. Wiesbaden: Harrassowitz.

Ghalioungui, P. 1963. *Magic and Medical Science in Ancient Egypt*. London: Hodder and Stoughton.

———. 1973. *The House of Life, Per-Ankh: Magic and Medical Science in Ancient Egypt*. 2nd ed. Amsterdam: B.M. Israël.

———. 1983. *The Physicians of Pharaonic Egypt*. Cairo: Al-Ahram Center for Scientific Translations.

———. 1987. *The Ebers Papyrus: A New English Translation, Commentaries, and Glossaries*. Cairo: Academy of Scientific Research and Technology.

Ghalioungui, P., and Z. el-Dawakhly. 1965. *Health and Healing in Ancient Egypt: A Pictorial Essay*. Cairo: Dar al-Maaref.

Ghalioungui, P., S. Khalil, and A.R. Ammar. 1963. "On an Ancient Egyptian Method of Diagnosing Pregnancy and Determining Foetal Sex." *Medical Historian* 7: 241–46.

Goelet, O., Jr. 1994. *The Egyptian Book of the Dead: The Book of Going Forth by Day*. San Francisco: Chronicle Books.

Grapow, H. 1954. *Anatomie und Physiologie.* Grundriss der Medizin der alten Ägypter I. Berlin: Akademie-Verlag.

———. 1955: *Von den medizinischen Texte.* Grundriss der Medizin der alten Ägypter II. Berlin: Akademie-Verlag.

———. 1956. *Kranker, Krankheiten und Arzt.* Grundriss der Medizin der alten Ägypter III. Berlin: Akademie-Verlag.

———. 1958. *Die medizinischen Texte in hieroglyphischer Umschreibung autographiert.* Grundriss der Medizin der alten Ägypter V. Berlin: Akademie-Verlag.

Griffith, F.Ll. 1898. *Hieratic Papyri from Kahun and Gurob (principally of the Middle Kingdom) I–II.* London: Bernard Quaritch.

Grunert, S. 2002. "Nicht nur sauber, sondern rein. Rituelle Reinigungsanweisungen aus dem Grab des Anchmahor in Saqqara." *Studien zur altägyptischen Kultur* 30: 137–51.

Hannig, R. 1997. *Die Sprache der Pharaonen. Großes Handwörterbuch Ägyptisch–Deutsch (2800–950 v.Chr.).* Mainz: Philipp von Zabern.

Harer, W.B. 1994. "Peseshkef: The First Special-Purpose Surgical Instrument." *Obstetrics and Gynecology* 83: 1053–55.

Hassan, S. 1932. *The Egyptian University Excavations at Giza (1929–1930).* Oxford: Oxford University Press.

Helck, W. 1971. *Das Bier im alten Ägypten.* Berlin: Gesellschaft für die Geschichte und Bibliographie des Brauwesens e.V., Institut für Gärungsgewerbe und Biotechnologie.

Hofmann, T. 2008. "Honig als 'Specificum': pEdwin Smith und die moderne Medizin." *Zeitschrift für ägyptische Sprache und Altertumskunde* 135: 40–49.

Houlihan, P.F. 1996. *The Animal World of the Pharaohs.* Cairo: American University in Cairo Press.

Iversen, E. 1939. *Papyrus Carlsberg No. VIII: With Some Remarks on the Egyptian Origin of Some Popular Birth Prognoses.* Det Kgl. Danske Videnskabernes Selskab, Historisk-filologiske Meddelelser, vol. XXV I, no. 5. Copenhagen: Ejnar Munksgaard.

James, T.G.H. 1953. *The Mastaba of Khentika Called Ikhekhi.* Memoir 30. Archaeological Survey of Egypt. London: Quaritch.

Janák, J. 2005. *Brána nebes. Bohové a démoni starého Egypta* [Heaven's Gate: Gods and Demons in Ancient Egypt]. Prague: Libri.

Joachim, H. 1890. *Papyros Ebers: Das älteste Buch über Heilkunde.* Berlin: Georg Reimer.

Jonckheere, F. 1947. *Le papyrus médical Chester Beatty.* Brussels: Fondation égyptologique Reine Élizabeth.

Kamal, H. 1967. *Dictionary of Pharaonic Medicine*. Cairo: National Publication House.

Kobilková, J., J.E. Jirásek, A. Martan, J. Mašata, and J. Živný. 2005. *Základy gynekologie a porodnictví* [The Essentials of Gynecology and Obstetrics]. Prague: Galén–Karolinum.

Kolta, K., and D. Schwarzmann-Schafhauser. 2000. *Die Heilkunde im alten Aegypten: Magie und Ratio in der Krankheitsvorstellung und therapeutischen Praxis*. Sudhoffs Archiv, Zeitschrift für Wissenschaftsgeschichte 42. Stuttgart: Franz Steiner Verlag.

Künzl, E. 1983. *Medizinische Instrumente aus Sepukralfunden der römischen Kaiserzeit*. Cologne: Rheinland Verlag.

Leca, A.P. 1971. *La médecine égyptienne au temps des Pharaons*. Paris: Dacosta.

————. 1976. *Les momies*. Paris: Hachette.

Leitz, Ch. 2000. "Die medizinischen Texte aus dem Alten Ägypten." In *Heilkunde und Hochkultur*, edited by A. Karenberg and Ch. Leitz, vol. 1, 17–33. Münster: LIT Verlag.

Lexa, F. 1923. *Staroegyptské čarodějnictví I–II* [Ancient Egyptian Magic]. Prague: Sfinx.

————. 1925. *La magie dans l'Égypte antique de l'Ancien Empire jusqu'à l'époque copte*. Paris: P. Geuthner.

Lexa, F., and A. Jirásek. 1941. "Papyrus Edwina Smitha [Edwin Smith Papyrus]." *Rozhledy v chirurgii* 20: 79–82, 107–109, 145–47, 169–72, 227–28, 286–90.

Lichtheim, M. 1976. *Ancient Egyptian Literature. Volume 2: The New Kingdom*. Berkeley, Los Angeles, and London: University of California Press.

Macků, F., and E. Čech. 2002. *Gynekologie* [Gynecology]. Prague: Informatorium.

Majno, G. 1975. *The Healing Hand: Man and Wound in the Ancient World*. Cambridge, MA: Harvard University Press.

Manniche, L. 1999. *An Ancient Egyptian Herbal*. 2nd ed. London: British Museum Press.

————. 2000. *Starověký egyptský herbář* [Ancient Egyptian Herbal]. Prague: Volvox Globator.

Martin, G.T. 1989. *The Royal Tomb at El-Amarna II. The Reliefs, Inscriptions, and Architecture*. The Rock Tombs of El-Amarna VII. Archaeological Survey of Egypt, Memoir 39. London: Egypt Exploration Society.

Matiegková, L. 1937. *Dítě v starém Egyptě* [The Child in Ancient Egypt]. Prague: Antropologický ústav Karlovy university v Praze.

Meyerhof, M. 1931. "Über den Papyrus Edwin Smith, das älteste Chirurgiebuch der Welt." *Zeitschrift für Chirurgie* 231: 645–90.

Miller, R.L. 1989. "Dqr, Spinning and Treatment of Guinea Worm in p.Ebers 865." *Journal of Egyptian Archaeology* 75: 249–54.

Naville, E. 1896. *The Temple of Deir el-Bahari II. Plates XXV–LV. The Ebony Shrine. Northern Half of the Middle Platform.* London: Egypt Exploration Fund.

Néret, G. 2001. *Napoleon and the Pharaohs: Description of Egypt.* Cologne: Taschen.

Nerlich, A.G., A. Zink, U. Szeimies, and H.G. Hagedorn. 2000. "Ancient Egyptian Prosthesis of the Big Toe." *Lancet* 356: 2176–79.

Nunn, J.F. 1996. *Ancient Egyptian Medicine.* London: British Museum Press.

Pahl, W.M. 1985–86. "Schädel-Hirn-Traumata im Alten Ägypten und ihre Therapie nach dem 'Wundenbuch' des Papyrus E. Smith (ca. 1500 v.Chr.)." *Ossa* 12: 93–131.

———. 1993. *Altägyptische Schädelchirurgie.* Stuttgart: G. Fischer.

Parkinson, R., and S. Quirke. 1995. *Papyrus.* Egyptian Bookshelf. London: British Museum Press.

Petrie, W.M.F. 1897. *Deshasheh.* Memoir of the Egypt Exploration Fund 15. London: Trübner.

Picardo, N.S. 2010. "(Ad)dressing Washptah: Illness or Injury in the Vizier's Death, as Related in His Tomb Biography." In *Millions of Jubilees: Studies in Honor of David P. Silverman, II,* edited by Z. Hawass and J. Houser Wegner, 94–104. Cairo: Conseil Suprême des Antiquités de l'Égypte.

Pliny the Elder. 1921–32. *Natural History.* Translated by H. Rackham. London: Heinemann.

Quack, F.J. 2003. "Methoden und Möglichkeiten der Erforschung der Medizin im Alten Ägypten." *Medizinhistorisches Journal* 38: 3–15.

Reeves, C. 1992. *Ancient Egyptian Medicine.* Shire Egyptology 15. Risborough: Shire Publications.

Reisner, G.A. 1905. *The Hearst Medical Papyrus.* Leipzig: J.C. Hinrichs.

Riddle, J.M. 1992. *Contraception and Abortion from the Ancient World to the Renaissance.* Cambridge, MA: Harvard University Press.

Robins, G. 1993. *Women in Ancient Egypt.* London: British Museum Press.

Rösing, F.W. 1980. "Medical Papyri and Medical Treatment—a Contradiction." *Antropologia contemporanea* 3: 1–7.

Roth, A.M. 1992. "The *psš-kf* and the 'Opening of the Mouth' Ceremony: A Ritual of Birth and Rebirth." *Journal of Egyptian Archaeology* 78: 113–47.

Scholl, R. 2002. *Der Papyrus Ebers. Die größte Buchrolle zur Heilkunde Altägyptens.* Schriften aus der Universitätsbibliothek 7. Leipzig: Universitätsbibliothek.

Schott, H. 1993. *Die Chronik der Medizin.* Harenberg: Chronik Verlag.

Simpson, W.K., ed. 2003. *The Literature of Ancient Egypt: An Anthology of Stories, Instructions, Stelae, Autobiographies, and Poetry.* Cairo: American University in Cairo Press.

Smith, G.E. 1908. "The Most Ancient Splints." *British Medical Journal* 28: 732–34.

———. 1912. *The Royal Mummies.* Catalogue général des antiquités égyptiennes du Musée du Caire (Nr. 61051–61100). Cairo: Institut français d'archéologie orientale.

Smith, G.E., and W.R. Dawson. 1924. *Egyptian Mummies.* London: G. Allen and Unwin.

Spigelman, M. 1997. "The Circumcision Scene in the Tomb of Ankhmahor: the First Record of Emergency Surgery?" *Bulletin of the Australian Centre for Egyptology* 8: 91–100.

Stephan, J. 2001. "Ordnungssysteme in der altägyptischen Medizin und ihre Überlieferung in den Europäischen Kulturkreis." Doctoral diss., Hamburg Universität.

Stevens, J.M. 1975. "Gynaecology from Ancient Egypt: The Papyrus Kahun: A Translation of the Oldest Treatise on Gynaecology That Has Survived the Ancient World." *Medical Journal of Australia* 21: 949–52.

Strouhal, E. 1980. "Folk Medical Treatment in Egyptian Nubians." In *Actas II Symposium de Antropología Biológica de España*, 363–76. Oviedo: Sociedad Española de Antropología Biológica.

———. 1981. "Folk Medical Treatment in Egyptian Nubians." *Annals of the Náprstek Museum Prague* 10: 183–93.

———. 1992a. *Life in Ancient Egypt.* Cambridge: Cambridge University Press.

———. 1992b. *Life of the Ancient Egyptians.* Norman, OK: Oklahoma University Press.

———. 1992c. *Life of the Ancient Egyptians.* Cairo: American University in Cairo Press.

———. 1994. "Tod und Mumifikation der alten Ägypter." *Mitteilungen der Berliner Gesellschaft für Anthropologie, Ethnologie und Urgeschichte* 15: 15–23.

———. 1999. "Ancient Egypt and Tuberculosis." In *Tuberculosis Past and Present*, edited by G. Pálfi, O. Dutour, and I. Hutás. Szeged: Golden Books Publications and Tuberculosis Foundation, 451–60.

———. 2002. "Nemoci a jejich léčení ve starém Egyptě" [Illnesses and Their Treatment in Ancient Egypt]. *Dějiny věd a techniky* 35: 3–4, 129–49.

———. 2005. "Staroegyptské lékařství" [Ancient Egyptian Medicine]. In *Kapitoly z dějin lékařství. Učební texty UK*, edited by M. Říhová, 15–25. Prague: Karolinum.

———. 2006a. "Smithův lékařský papyrus a nález jednoho z jeho případů" [Smith Medical Papyrus and the Discovery of One of Its Cases]. *Zdravotnické noviny* 55, no. 29–30: 10–11.

———. 2006b. "Historie nádorů ve starověku podle písemných dokladů" [The History of Tumors in Antiquity According to the Written Documents]. In *Historia—Medicina—Cultura. Sborník k dějinám mediciny,* edited by K. Černý and P. Svobodný, 19–33. Prague: Karolinum.

———. 2007a. "Anthropology of the Egyptian Nubian Men." *Anthropologie* 45, no. 2–3: 148–51.

———. 2007b. "Tracce di variola epidemico nelle famiglia di Ramesse V della XX dinastia egiziana." In *Il terribile vento flagelli epidemic,* edited by G. Baggieri and M. Di Giacomo, 93–99. Rome: Melami.

———. 2008. *The Memphite Tomb of Horemheb, Commander-in-chief of Tutankhamun IV: Human Skeletal Remains.* Egypt Exploration Society Excavation Memoir 87. London: Egypt Exploration Society.

Strouhal, E., and L. Bareš. 1993. *Secondary Cemetery in the Mastaba of Ptahshepses at Abusir.* Prague: Czechoslovak Institute of Egyptology, Charles University, Prague.

Strouhal, E., and L. Horáčková. 2007. "A Trauma of Cervical Spine Described in the Edwin Smith Papyrus Found in a Ptolemaic Tomb at Saqqara." *Études et travaux* 21: 129–37.

Strouhal, E., and J. Jungwirth. 1981. "Künstliche Eingriffe an Schädeln aus den Spätrömischen bis Frühbyzantinischen Gräberfeldern in Sayala (Ägyptisch-Nubien)." *Anthropologie* 19, no. 2: 149–60.

Strouhal, E., and A. Němečková. 2004. "Paleopathological Find of a Sacral Neurilemmoma from Ancient Egypt." *American Journal of Physical Anthropology* 125, no. 4: 320–28.

———. 2008. *Trpěli i dávní lidé nádory? Historie a paleopatologie nádorů, zvláště zhoubných* [Did Past People Also Suffer from Tumors? A History and Paleopathology of Tumours, Particularly Malignant Ones.] Prague: Karolinum.

———. 2009. "Velké defekty v lebeční klenbě u lidí v minulosti" [Big Defects in the Cranial Vaults of Past People]. *Pohybové ústrojí* 16, no. 1–2: 31–43.

Strudwick, N.C. 2005. *Texts from the Pyramid Age.* Atlanta: Society of Biblical Literature.

Sullivan, R. 1996. "The Identity and Work of the Ancient Egyptian Surgeon." *Journal of the Royal Society of Medicine* 89: 467–73.

———. 1997. "Divine and Rational: The Reproductive Health of Women in Ancient Egypt." CME Review Article 28. *Obstetrical and Gynecological Survey* 52, no. 10: 635–42.

———. 1998. "Proto-surgery in Ancient Egypt." *Acta Medica (Hradec Králové)* 41: 109–20.

Thompson, R.C. 1923. *Assyrian Medical Texts*. London: Trustees of the British Museum.

Vachala, B. 1992. *Moudrost starého Egypta* [The Wisdom of Ancient Egypt]. Prague: KPK.

———. 1994. *Pověsti a legendy faraonského Egypta* [Tales and Legends of Pharaonic Egypt]. Prague: KPK.

———. 2005. "Ani princezna Meketaton nepřišla. Tajemství rodiny faraona Achnatona trvají" [Not Even Princess Meketaten Came: Secrets of the Family of Pharaoh Akhenaten Continue]. *Vesmír* 84: 340–43.

———. 2006. "Tabulky posvátných olejů z jižního Abúsíru (Egypt)" [Sacred Oil Tablets from Abusir South (Egypt)]. In *Ve službách archeologie VII. Sborník věnovaný 85. narozeninám Doc. PhDr. Karla Valocha, DrSc*, edited by V. Hašek, R. Nekuda, and M. Ruttkay, 465–71. Brno: Muzejní a vlastivědná společnost.

———. 2007a. "Obřízka ve starém Egyptě. Ikonografické a textové doklady" [Circumcision in Ancient Egypt: Iconographic and Textual Evidence.]. *Vesmír* 86: 660–64.

———. 2007b. "Starověký Egypt" [Ancient Egypt]. In *Kruh prstenu. Světové dějiny sexuality, erotiky a lásky od počátku do současnosti I* [The Circle of the Ring: The World History of Sexuality, Eroticism, and Love from the Beginnings up to the Present Day, I], edited by J. Malina et al., 421–67. Brno: Akademické nakladatelství CERM.

———. 2009. *Staroegyptská Kniha mrtvých (Překlad)* [Ancient Egyptian Book of the Dead (Translation)]. Prague: Dokořán.

Vachala, B., and J. Svoboda. 1989. "Die Steinmesser aus Abusir. Ein Artefakt aus der Sicht von zwei historischen Disziplinen." *Zeitschrift für ägyptische Sprache und Altertumskunde* 116: 174–81.

Veiga, P.A. da Silva. 2009. *Health and Medicine in Ancient Egypt: Magic and Science*. BAR International Series 1967. Oxford: Archaeopress.

von Deines, H., and H. Grapow. 1959. *Wörterbuch der ägyptischen Drogennamen*. Grundriss der Medizin der alten Ägypter VI. Berlin: Akademie Verlag.

von Deines, H., H. Grapow, and W. Westendorf. 1958. *Übersetzung der medizinischen Texte*. Grundriss der Medizin der alten Ägypter IV, nos. 1–2. Berlin: Akademie Verlag.

von Deines, H., and W. Westendorf. 1957. *Zur ägyptischen Wortforschung V. Proben aus den Wörterbüchern zu den medizinischen Texten*. Abhandlungen der Deutschen Akademie der Wissenschaften zu Berlin. Berlin: Akademie Verlag.

———. 1961. *Wörterbuch der medizinischen Texte*. Grundriss der Medizin der alten Ägypter VII, nos. 1–2. Berlin: Akademie Verlag.

———. 1962. *Grammatik der medizinischen Texte*. Grundriss der Medizin der alten Ägypter VIII. Berlin: Akademie Verlag.

Voß, S. 2009. "Ludwig Borchardt's Recherche zur Herkunft des pEbers." *MDAIK* 65: 373–76.

Verner, M., L. Bareš, and B. Vachala. 1998. *Ilustrovaná encyklopedie starého Egypta* [An Illustrated Encyclopaedia of Ancient Egypt]. Prague: Karolinum.

Vymazalová, H. 2006. *Staroegyptská matematika. Hieratické matematické texty* [Ancient Egyptian Mathematics: Hieratic Mathematical Texts]. Dějiny matematiky 31. Prague: Český egyptologický ústav Filozofické fakulty Univerzity Karlovy v Praze—Jednota českých matematiků a fyziků.

Waltari, M. 1949. *The Egyptian*. New York: G.P. Putnam's Sons.

Watterson, B. 1991. *Women in Ancient Egypt*. New York: Alan Sutton, Stroud, St. Martin's Press.

Weeks, K.R. 1970. "The Anatomical Knowledge of the Ancient Egyptians and the Representation of the Human Figure in Egyptian Art." Doctoral diss., Yale University.

Wegner, J. 2002. "A Decorated Birth-brick from South Abydos." *Egyptian Archaeology* 21: 3–4.

———. 2009. "A Decorated Birth-brick from South Abydos: New Evidence on Childbirth and Birth Magic in the Middle Kingdom." In *Archaism and Innovation: Studies in the Culture of Middle Kingdom Egypt*, edited by D.P. Silverman, W.K. Simpson, and J. Wegner, 447–96. New Haven: Department of Near Eastern Languages and Civilizations, Yale University; Philadelphia: University of Pennsylvania Museum of Archaeology and Anthropology.

Westendorf, W. 1959. *Wörterbuch der ägyptischen Drogennamen* (Grundriss der Medizin der alten Ägypter VI). Berlin: Akademie Verlag.

———. 1966. *Papyrus Edwin Smith. Ein medizinisches Lehrbuch aus dem Alten Ägypten*. Bern: Hans Huber.

———. 1992. *Erwachen der Heilkunst. Die Medizin im Alten Ägypten.* Zürich: Artemis & Winkler.

———. 1999. *Handbuch der altägyptischen Medizin.* Handbuch der Orientalistik 36. Leiden: Brill.

Wildung, D. 1994. *Egyptian Art in Berlin: Masterpieces in the Bodenmuseum and in Charlottenburg.* Mainz am Rhein: Philipp von Zabern.

Wilkinson, R.H. 2003. *The Complete Gods and Goddesses of Ancient Egypt.* Cairo: American University in Cairo Press.

Wreszinski, W. 1909. *Der grosse medizinische Papyrus des Berliner Museums (Pap. Berl. 3038) in Facsimile und Umschrift mit Übersetzung, Kommentar und Glossar.* Leipzig: J.C. Hinrichs.

———. 1912. *Der Londoner medizinische Papyrus (Brit. Museum Nr. 10059) und der Papyrus Hearst in Transcription, Übersetzung und Kommentar.* Leipzig: J.C. Hinrichs.

———. 1913. *Der Papyrus Ebers, Umschrift, Übersetzung und Kommentar I–II.* Leipzig: J.C. Hinrichs.

———. 1923. *Atlas zur Altägyptischen Kulturgeschichte.* Leipzig: J.C. Hinrichs.

Yamazaki, N. 2003. *Zaubersprüche für Mutter und Kind. Papyrus Berlin 3027.* Achet Schriften zur Ägyptologie B2. Berlin: Achet Verlag.

Žába, Z. 1968. *Tesáno do kamene, psáno na papyrus* [Carved in Stone, Written on Papyrus]. Prague: Svoboda.

INDEX

Nut 113, 114, 129, 130, 134, 176, 196
nuts, pine 105, 108, 109, 143, 144, 150

ochre 45, 104, 118, 120, 121, 126, 146,
    181, 185
oil 26, 27, 28, 29, 30, 31, 33, 34, 35, 36,
    37, 38, 40, 41, 42, 43, 44, 46, 47,
    48, 49, 52, 53, 55, 57, 60, 61, 62,
    64, 66, 68, 69, 73, 74, 76, 78, 80,
    92, 102, 105, 106, 108, 109, 115,
    116, 117, 118, 119, 121, 122, 123,
    126, 143, 144, 145, 148, 149, 150,
    151, 152, 153, 156, 158, 161, 174,
    175, 176, 177, 179, 193, 196, 202;
    fresh 106, 107, 109, 110, 111,
    127, 161, 180; white 106, 121
onion 105, 111, 122, 125, 128, 149,
    162, 199
opening of the mouth ritual 87
operation (surgery) 80, 81, 83, 86, 87,
    89, 91, 92, 94, 95, 136
opium 91
Osiris 33, 113, 115, 129, 134, 139, 191,
    193
ostrich 75; eggs 33, 60, 130
ovulation 141, 147

pain (ache) 25, 29, 31, 40, 44, 45, 47,
    55, 57, 63, 64, 65, 66, 68, 69, 70,
    71, 72, 73, 89, 91, 92, 98, 103,
    107, 108, 109, 110, 112, 114,
    115, 120, 121, 123, 125, 132,
    140, 141, 142, 143, 144, 145,
    146, 149, 150, 152, 162, 169,
    173, 174, 175, 176, 180, 182,
    183, 185, 188, 195, 197, 199;
    menstrual 147; relief 90
pakh, bird 113
pakh-seryt, plant 105, 122, 149
palliative care 55, 54, 68, 92
palm 32, 33, 59, 110, 127, 180; tree
    105, 110, 145
papyrus, ingredient 104, 106, 116, 131,
    197

papyrus, production 3
paralysis 59, 66, 68, 130, 199
parasitic disease 9, 195
Passalacqua, Giuseppe 16
pea 122, 149
pellitory (Spanish chamomile) 63, 104,
    116, 153
perch, Nile 193, 199
Persea 105
Peseshet 139
peseshkef (knife) 87, 88
Petrie, Flinders 12
Philae x, 155
physician 1, 2, 6, 8, 10, 13, 23, 27, 33,
    53, 54, 56, 57, 60, 61, 64, 68, 69,
    70, 72, 73, 75, 76, 77, 78, 79, 81,
    82, 84, 85, 86, 88, 92, 143, 144,
    145, 148, 161, 162, 163, 172;
    medical specializations 2, 8, 80–
    84, 136, 138–39, 172
placenta 106, 110, 115, 117, 170, 172,
    174, 179, 180, 181, 189
plague 79
Pliny the Elder 2
poppy 26, 44, 47, 71, 90, 91, 104, 116,
    197
potamogeton 104, 122, 179
pregnancy ix, 16, 17, 97, 98, 99, 101,
    142, 147, 148, 156, 161, 164,
    165–67, 168, 171, 172, 173, 184;
    extrauterine 156; tests 99, 158–65
pubic region 107, 108, 109, 114, 117,
    120, 122, 129, 139, 142, 143,
    145, 146, 147, 149, 151, 180,
    184, 198, 199
puerperium 101
pulse 27, 54, 57, 161, 163
pumice 25, 44, 71
Pyramid Texts 80, 205

Qubbat el-Hawa x, 93,
Quibell, James Edward 12
Qur'an 7, 191
Qur'anic schools 7